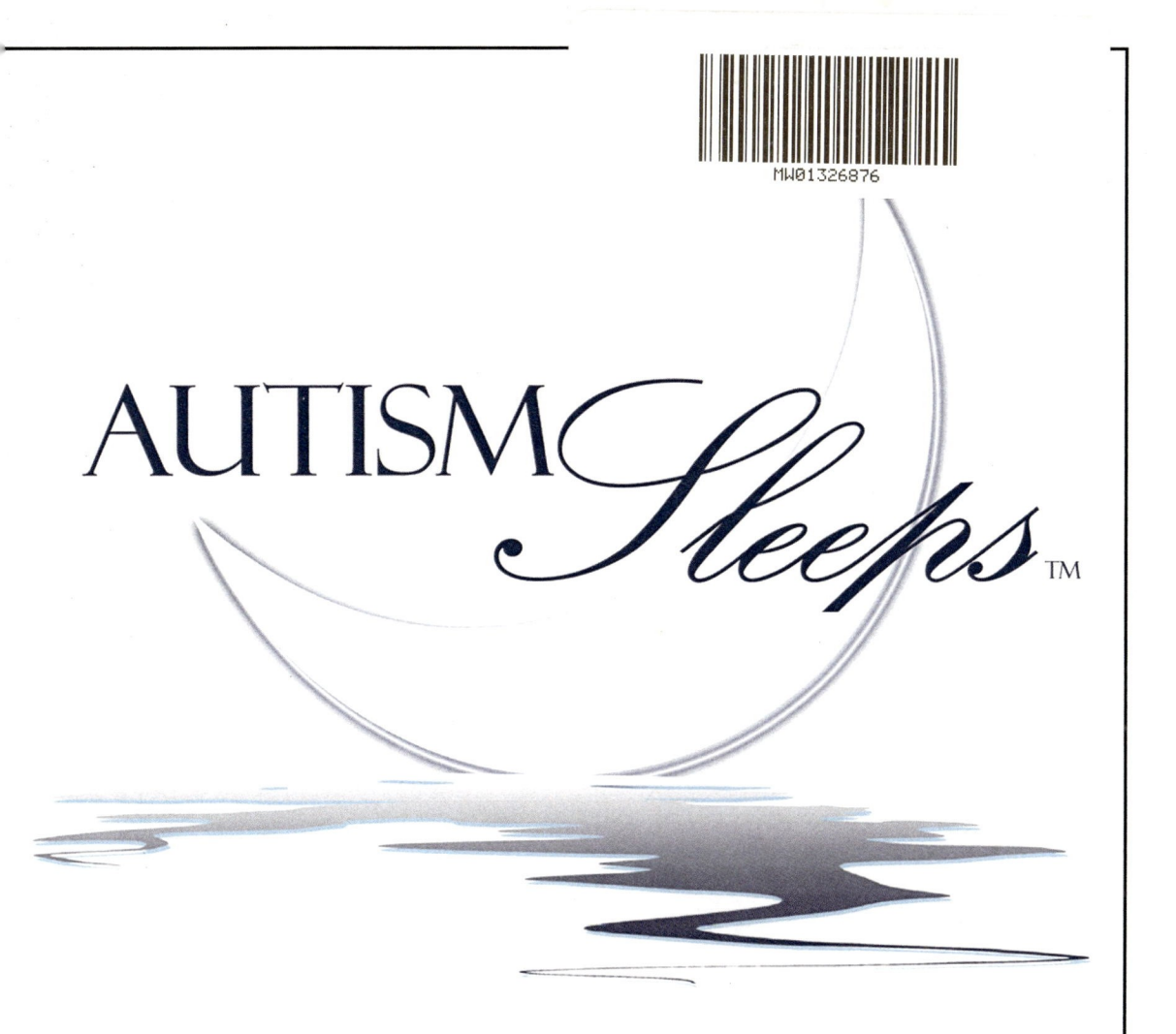

AUTISM *Sleeps* ™

Sensory Strategies to Help Restless Minds Sleep!

Ileana S. McCaigue
Occupational Therapist & Wellness Consultant

DISCLAIMER

The information in this book may be used with persons of all ages. However, it is recommended that each child or adolescent with whom this book is to be implemented should be evaluated regarding his or her general level of sensory processing abilities prior to beginning the use of sensory strategies. This is done in order to determine the sensory area(s) where the child or adolescent is most likely to respond favorably to the strategies used.

The sensory strategies listed in this manual are examples of possible solutions for persons who suffer from sleep problems. Many of them have proven to be successful in this author's past experiences with children, adolescents and adults who had difficulty either getting to sleep or staying asleep as a result of sensory processing concerns that may or may not have been formally identified.

The author is not responsible for any possible injuries, sensory reactions or accidents that may arise out of the use or misuse of the materials listed in this book. It is further presumed that if an assessment is needed, the caregiver has sought the expertise of a therapist that is trained in the signs of sensory processing disorders, as well as those of sensory overload, and who could identify areas of possible oversensitivities or need in order to implement safety precautions when utilizing these suggested strategies. Physical limitations may also prevent the use of some activities that may be contraindicated, depending on the individual's abilities/disabilities. Use of equipment listed and the sensory strategies suggested should be done only after reading the possible sensory overreactions that could occur and should be done under parental supervision in the case of a minor. Additional assistance by a **trained and specialized therapist** or other provider is recommended should a more delineated plan be needed.

ISBN 978-0-615-86017-6

Copyright © 2013, Ileana S. McCaigue, OTR/L

Edited by Leslie G. Champion

Cover and Logo Designed by Poseygraphics.com

For additional information contact:

Handy O. T. Treatment Tools, LLC

P. O. Box 1658, Suwanee, Georgia 30024

Email: ileana@HOTRxTools.com

Websites: www.HOTRxTools.com
            www.NIKKEN.com/SensoryTools4U

TABLE OF CONTENTS

TABLE OF CONTENTS—(Continued)

DEDICATION

This book is dedicated to Dr. Amy Lang who was the first physician and orthopedist to introduce me to wellness interventions, specifically the use of magnetic products and Acupuncture, and the role they can play in our daily lives to reduce discomfort and improve daily function.

It is also dedicated to the parents of the many children, adolescents and adults with Autism Spectrum Disorder and other Sensory Processing Disorders with whom I have worked that could not concentrate at school or in the community partly from not being able get a much needed full night's sleep. There are many in our schools with this difficulty...those that are students with special needs, as well as staff and those children that are more typical.

My hope is that the sensory sleep strategies described herein will be able to help at least one individual in each home to enable that person and those that live with him or her to benefit from the healing effects of healthy sleep!

Ileana S. McCaigue, OTR/L

ACKNOWLEDGMENTS

Appreciation is expressed to the parents of the individuals discussed in the case studies (Brenda and Brian, Angela and Mike Land, Claire and Mark Dees) for allowing me to share with others the many sensory strategies that worked to help their special needs child sleep.

Thanks are given to Vickie Johnson and Brandy Posey for their artistic guidance and design assistance, Jodi Pierce for her publishing and publicity advice, Leslie Champion for her editing and photographic permit assistance, and to the reviewers who provided their valuable time to read and critique this book. In addition, thanks are given to Sheri and Jack Clarke who helped me attain deep, continuous and restful sleep through education and training on the use of holistic products. These items proved to be the vital solutions that enabled me to benefit from the quantity and quality of sleep needed to be at my daily best.

SPECIAL THANKS

Special thanks are given to my son, Ryan; my sister, Vivian Gammell; my dear friend, Cindy Demme; and the rest of my family and friends for their ongoing encouragement and support in completing this book.

Ileana S. McCaigue, OTR/L

INTRODUCTION

Having worked as a therapist in many settings since 1977, a common concern that I heard routinely was that the person with whom I was working had problems sleeping more than a few hours at a time. If he or she slept, often sleep was interrupted with early or frequent awakenings.

As a typically excellent sleeper, my own sleep/wake cycle was overturned after experiencing a near fatal automobile accident in 2002. I suffered several fractures, as well as a mild head injury where I lost my short-term memory for nine months, and was confined to a wheelchair for three months. So I understood very well how it felt to experience poor quality sleep, making it extremely challenging to get through the next day.

As a result of my head injury, I was diagnosed with a form of Narcolepsy, a sleep disorder, called Post Traumatic Hypersomnia. This is a condition in which I was functioning during my daytime activities while being in a state of constant shallow sleep, and at night never getting into a level of deeper, restful sleep to "recharge" my body for the next day. Therefore, I was either sleepy throughout the day or falling asleep during periods when I would be sitting still or even while driving in slow-moving traffic. Recognizing this as a potentially dangerous condition, I sought the medical advice of my very trusted internist who recommended that I have a 24-hour sleep study. Of course, I readily agreed and completed the study. The sleep specialist anticipated that I would exhibit a problem called Sleep Apnea where there would be periods when I would stop breathing during the night. However, the findings were surprising to him and me as well. While I slept throughout the night without any significant loss of oxygen of greater than 2-3 percent, I was in a state of deep sleep during every sleep cycle only for very brief periods of time or not at all. This was in 2004, and it was then that I began researching sleep and natural or sensory-based strategies that could help me to achieve healing, deep sleep and the return to a typical day-night or diurnal pattern without the need for chemicals.

This book is a compilation of what I learned about sleep to help myself, as well as those that I serve as an Occupational Therapist. The additional knowledge that I gained as a wellness consultant served to enhance the development of essential sensory strategies that became part of the approaches outlined in this resource. I hope these elements of nature and universal strategies will help others as much as they have helped me.

Ileana S. McCaigue, OTR/L

SELF QUIZ: Pre-Test Questions

Name: _____   Date: _____

1.   When do most children give up taking a nap?
      a.   2 years
      b.   3 years
      c.   4 years
      d.   5 years

2.   Which of the following might interfere with a child sleeping through the night?
      a.   falling asleep with a bottle
      b.   falling asleep on the couch and then being moved to the bed
      c.   falling asleep while watching TV
      d.   all of the above

3.   A good security object in bed as part of the routine could include a…
      a.   blanket
      b.   bottle of juice or milk
      c.   stuffed animal
      d.   either a or c

4.   How much sleep does a 3-month-old usually need?
      a.   20 hours
      b.   15 hours
      c.   12 hours
      d.   9 hours

5.   How much sleep does a 9-year-old need?
      a.   12 hours
      b.   11 hours
      c.   10 hours
      d.   9 hours

(CONTINUED ON NEXT PAGE)

SELF-QUIZ: Pre-Test Questions (Continued)-

Name: _____   Date: _____

6.   How much sleep does a 2-year-old usually need?
        a. 15 hours
        b. 13 hours
        c. 11 hours
        d. 9 hours

7.   How much sleep does a 14-year-old need?
        a. 11 hours
        b. 10 hours
        c. 9 hours
        d. 8 hours

8.   How much sleep does a 5-year-old need?
        a. 15 hours
        b. 13 hours
        c. 11 hours
        d. 9 hours

9.   Children with obstructive sleep apnea usually…
        a. snore
        b. snore loudly and have periods where they stop breathing
        c. are thin
        d. have had their tonsils taken out

10.   Not getting enough sleep at night can cause children to…
        a. have trouble paying attention
        b. have headaches
        c. be hyperactive
        d. all of the above

[END OF TEST]

PRE-TEST SCORE: _____% Correct

AUTISM SLEEPS

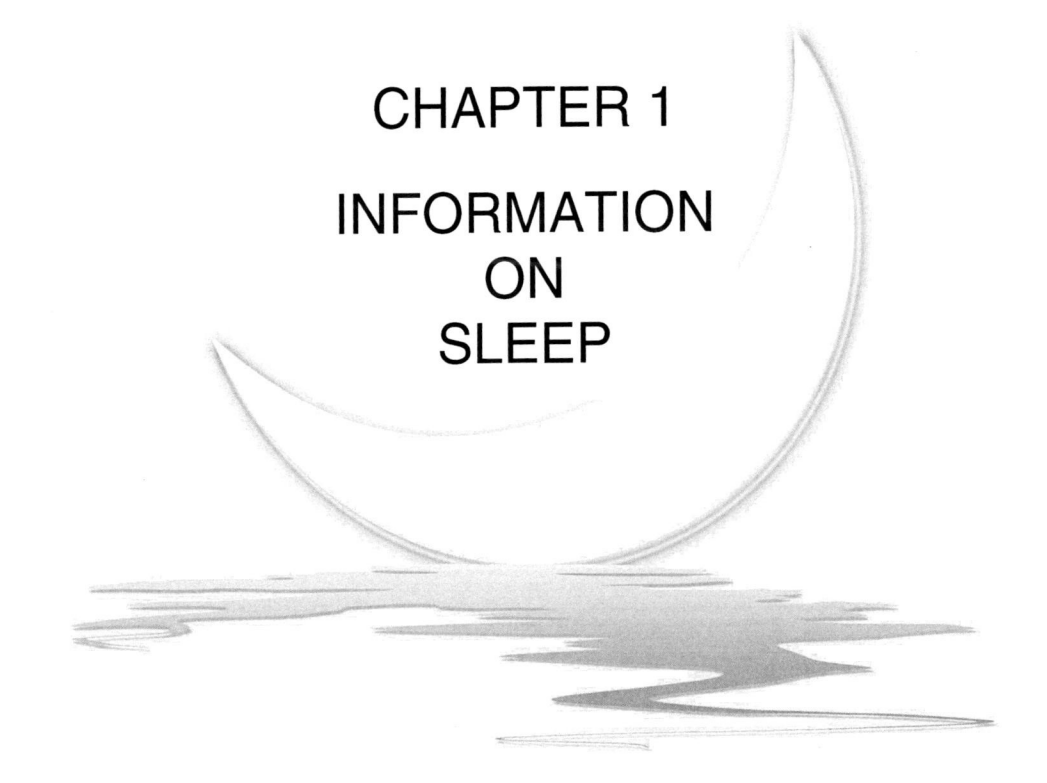

CHAPTER 1

INFORMATION ON SLEEP

AUTISM SLEEPS

More than ever…
Children are being diagnosed with

"neurobiological disorders" such as:

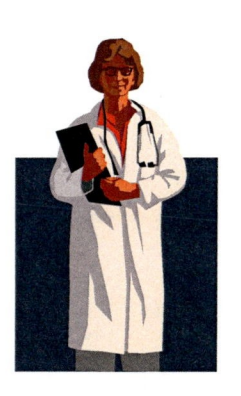

AUTISM SPECTRUM DISORDERS *[ASD]*:

Severe, Moderate, Mild or Asperger's Type;

BIPOLAR or MANIC-DEPRESSIVE

DISORDER;

CLINICAL DEPRESSION;

SENSORY-INTEGRATION

DISORDERS *[SID]*

or

SENSORY PROCESSING DISORDERS

[SPD] : Sensory Modulation, Discrimination

or Sensory-Based Motor Disorder

and/or

Neurobiological disorders: *(Continued)*—

ATTENTION-DEFICIT/ HYPERACTIVITY DISORDERS *[ADHD]*: Hyperactive, Inattentive or Combination Type.

Sleep difficulties usually accompany these disorders which, in turn, are aggravated by a lack of healthy sleep that can follow us into adulthood!

As a result of poor quality sleep, the activities required for daily living can be impacted as follow:

- Inability to awaken to begin a daily schedule;
- Irritability or erratic behavior to begin/continue throughout each day;
- Inability to demonstrate sustained attention to follow simple directions at home or school due to daytime sleepiness;
- Difficulty retaining new information learned due to interrupted nighttime when the daily activities are processed and integrated.

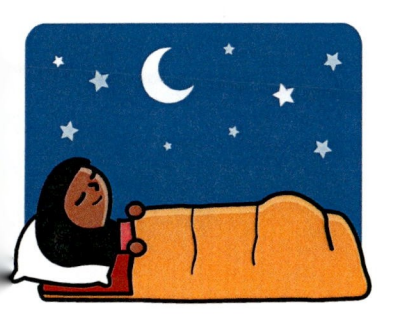

What happens during *sleep*?

William Shakespeare called *sleep...*
"nature's soft nurse".

Expert opinions vary, but sleep is believed to ...

→ "Recharge" our energy supplies like a cell phone

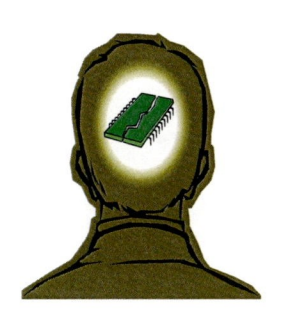

→ Repair body tissues through hormonal changes

→ Process and store memories to promote learning, optimizing brain functions

-and-

→ Be a critical component of health

SLEEP is...

1 of 3 THINGS

OUR BODIES CRAVE:

FOOD

SEX

SLEEP*

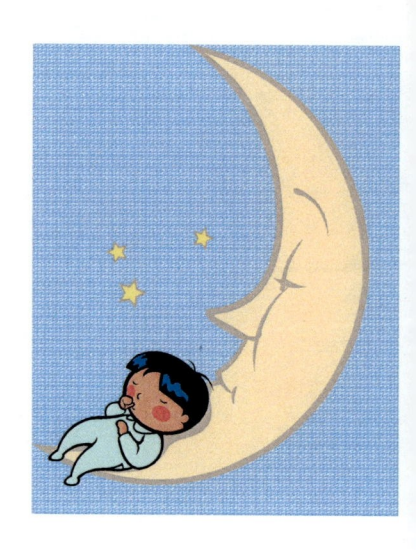

*If not enough sleep, our bodies crave food, specifically carbohydrates, which can cause weight gain and be one of the roots of childhood obesity. Through regular, better sleep, weight loss can result.

- Studies performed in 2010 indicated that children with persistent sleep problems are more likely to suffer from depression, anxiety, alcohol and drug abuse.

Types of *Sleep* **Patterns**:

Non-Rapid Eye Movements

or

"NREM"

[Stages 1-4]

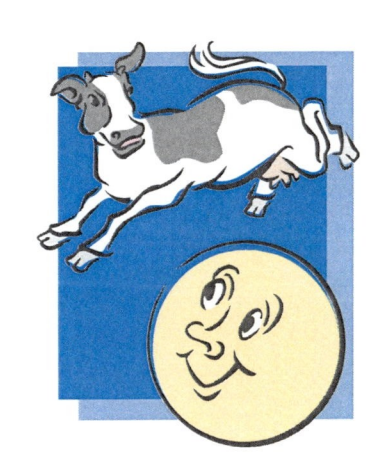

and

Rapid Eye Movements

or

"REM" SLEEP

[Stage 5]

What Are the
5 Stages of *Sleep*?

#1: **NREM**

This is a hazy, light sleep that is easily disrupted. It is usually less than 10 to 30 minutes to 2 hours in persons with difficulty for sleep onset.

#2: **NREM** (Continued)

Moderately light sleep occurs, but heart rate and brain waves are slower. The body temperature drops to prepare for deeper sleep. It is about 30 minutes of total sleep time.

#3: **NREM** (Continued)

It is difficult to differentiate physiologically from Stage 4; brain waves slow into *"Delta sleep"*.

What Are the
5 Stages of *Sleep*?

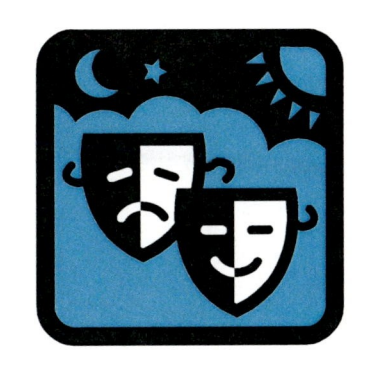

#4: <u>NREM</u> (Continued)

Stage 4 is deepest sleep, but close to
Stage 3 in a "dead sleep" or "out like a
light". It is very difficult to arouse. Most
of the body's repair work is done here.
This is usually when sleep terrors and
sleepwalking occur.

#5: <u>REM SLEEP</u>

The eyes flutter with back and forth motions.
Most vivid and prolonged dreams occur here.
The brain is most active, but the body is
temporarily paralyzed to not act out dreams.
Heart rate, metabolism, sexual arousal, blood
flow, brain activity and blood pressure increase

What Are the
5 Stages of *Sleep*?

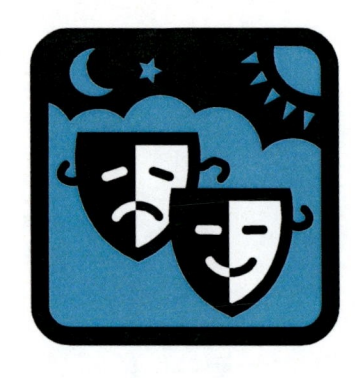

#5: <u>**REM SLEEP**</u> (Continued)

with erratic respiration. This is the important
stage for learning and memory processing.
Persons are more easily awakened from this
stage. It is usually about 20-25 percent of total
sleep time.

A Typical Sleep Cycle

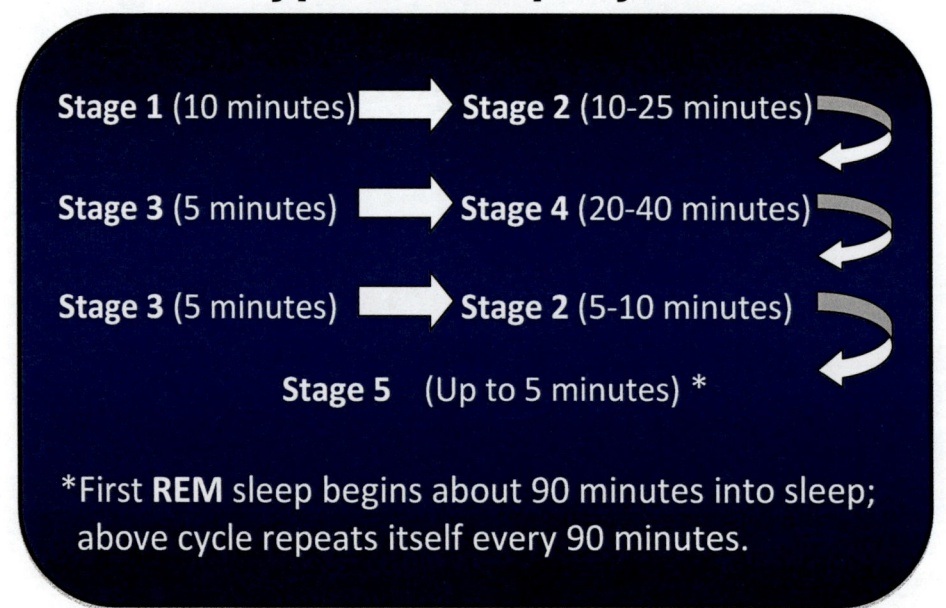

Stage 1 (10 minutes) ➡ **Stage 2** (10-25 minutes)

Stage 3 (5 minutes) ➡ **Stage 4** (20-40 minutes)

Stage 3 (5 minutes) ➡ **Stage 2** (5-10 minutes)

Stage 5 (Up to 5 minutes) *

*First **REM** sleep begins about 90 minutes into sleep;
above cycle repeats itself every 90 minutes.

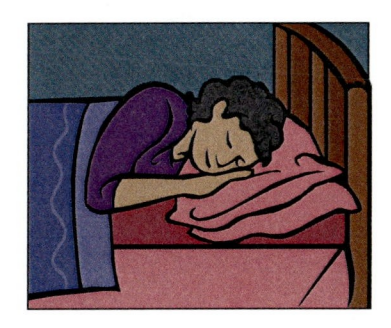

OUR SLEEP PATTERNS ...

change with age.

- Newborns through age 1 year go directly to REM sleep with shorter complete cycles of only 50-60 minutes on average.

- Stages 3 ("Delta" sleep) and 4 (deep sleep) last longer in young children which is why they are more difficult to arouse.

- 17 percent of children, as opposed to 4 percent of adults, sleepwalk with peak behavior at age 11-12 years.

- As we age, our nighttime awakenings increase. Typically this begins at age 40 with healthy sleepers; however, for those with poor sleep quality, it can occur at any age.

HOW BEDTIMES IMPACT OUR HEALTH...

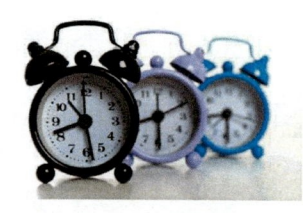

Deep or "Delta" sleep helps fight the effects of daily stress. It keeps our energy levels high and also helps to maintain steady weight. The center for deepest sleep in our brain is in the frontal lobe inside the skull at the forehead, above our eyes [designated by the lighted area below]. This is also the center for attention, alertness and decision-making skills which needs to be calmed or quieted in order to attain deep sleep.

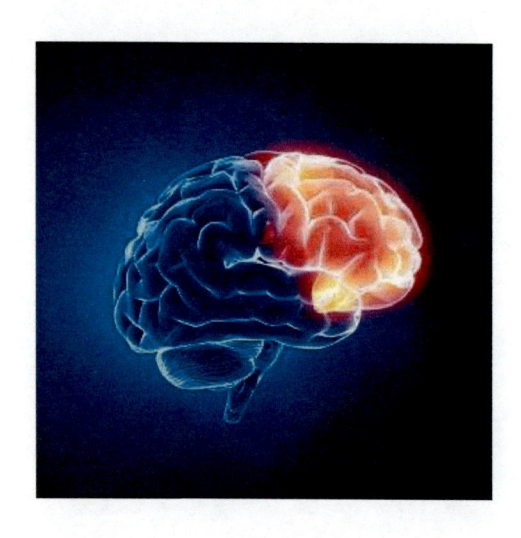

The deepest and most restorative or regenerative sleep occurs between the hours of *10:00 P.M. and 2:00 A.M.* Our sleep levels and our sleep cycle become more superficial after 2:00 A.M. If this occurs and you awaken between 2:00 and 3:00 A.M., it will be more difficult to return to a state of deep sleep. If you are

HOW BEDTIMES IMPACT OUR HEALTH... (Continued)—

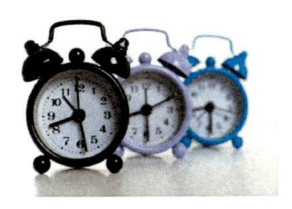

still awake after 10:00 P.M., then the *"second wind"* phenomenon occurs because there is a rise in Serotonin, a neurotransmitter that increases alertness. This causes increased energy and mental activity at that time.

If you stay awake after 10:00 P.M. to work on the computer, read or watch television, there is a continuation of light exposure. This light input goes through the eyes or *Optic Nerve* to the *Pineal Gland* in the middle, center area of the brain where our internal clock is housed in an area called the *Hippocampus*. This section also regulates appetite, body temperature and other biological states. [Depicted by the central blue area in the brain diagram.] Typically, the sunset is sensed through our biological or internal *"clock"* and helps the *Pineal Gland* secrete a very strong, nocturnal, antioxidant hormone, *Melatonin*, which helps us to feel drowsy and induces sleep. If bedtime is later than 10:00 P.M., it generally takes longer to fall

HOW BEDTIMES IMPACT OUR HEALTH...

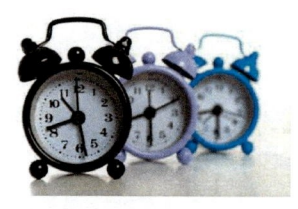

asleep due to the shift in the amount of light our eyes take in, causing an increase versus a decrease in mental energy.

Getting to sleep before 10:00 P.M. not only gives the body the added benefit of greater rest, but it also takes advantage of the body's natural neurochemistry to benefit from the deepest sleep levels. Adjusting bedtime from 11:00 to 10:00 P.M. would provide important benefits that would significantly impact the body's general health, especially regarding weight, levels of alertness during the next day, and overall physical and mental capabilities.

Effects

of

SLEEP

DEPRIVATION

- Irritability
- Cognitive impairment
- Memory lapses or loss
- Impaired moral judgement
- Severe yawning
- Hallucinations
- Symptoms similar to ADHD
- Impaired immune system
- Risk of diabetes Type 2

- Increased heart rate variability
- Risk of heart disease

- Increased reaction time
- Decreased accuracy
- Tremors
- Aches

Other:
- Growth suppression
- Risk of obesity
- Decreased temperature

HOW MUCH SLEEP DO CHILDREN, ADOLESCENTS & ADULTS NEED?

Recommendations According to the National Sleep Foundation:

- **NEWBORNS**   10.5 - 18 hours (0-2 months)
- **INFANTS**   11 - 15 hours   (3-11 months)
- **TODDLERS**   12 - 14 hours
- **PRESCHOOLERS**   11 - 13 hours   ← **69% of typical children have sleep problems**
- **SCHOOL-AGED**   10 - 11 hours

- **ADOLESCENTS & YOUNG ADULTS**   9 hours minimum

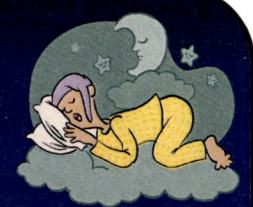

- **ADULTS**   8 hours a night on average

- **OLDER ADULTS**   7 hours   (Age 55-84)

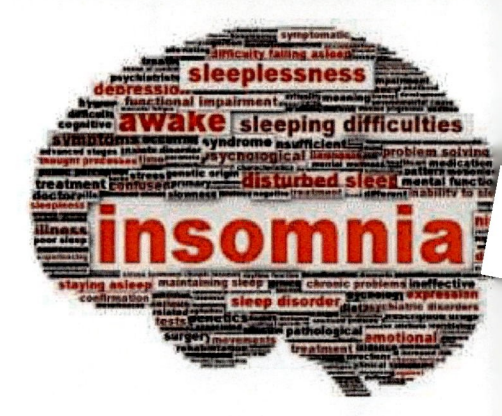

WHAT ARE COMMON
SLEEP DISORDERS?

- *NIGHTMARES*—During times of stress or change in routine and usually occur later in the night.

- *SLEEP TERRORS/SLEEPWALKING* —Mostly from 4-8 years of age and usually occur early in the night.

- *SLEEP APNEA* —Serious disorder with pauses in breathing; may snore loudly and be sleepy during daytime, especially with *Obstructive Sleep Apnea (OSA)*.

- *NARCOLEPSY* —Often first seen in puberty, but can occur as early as 10 years old as evidenced by excessive daytime sleepiness and uncontrollable "sleep attacks". A type can also be diagnosed as Post-Traumatic Hypersomnia after an acquired brain injury.

- *RESTLESS LEG SYNDROME*— Hereditary in 50 percent of persons and occurs possibly due to vitamin and iron deficiencies, nerve disorders, kidney failure or as a reaction to certain medications.

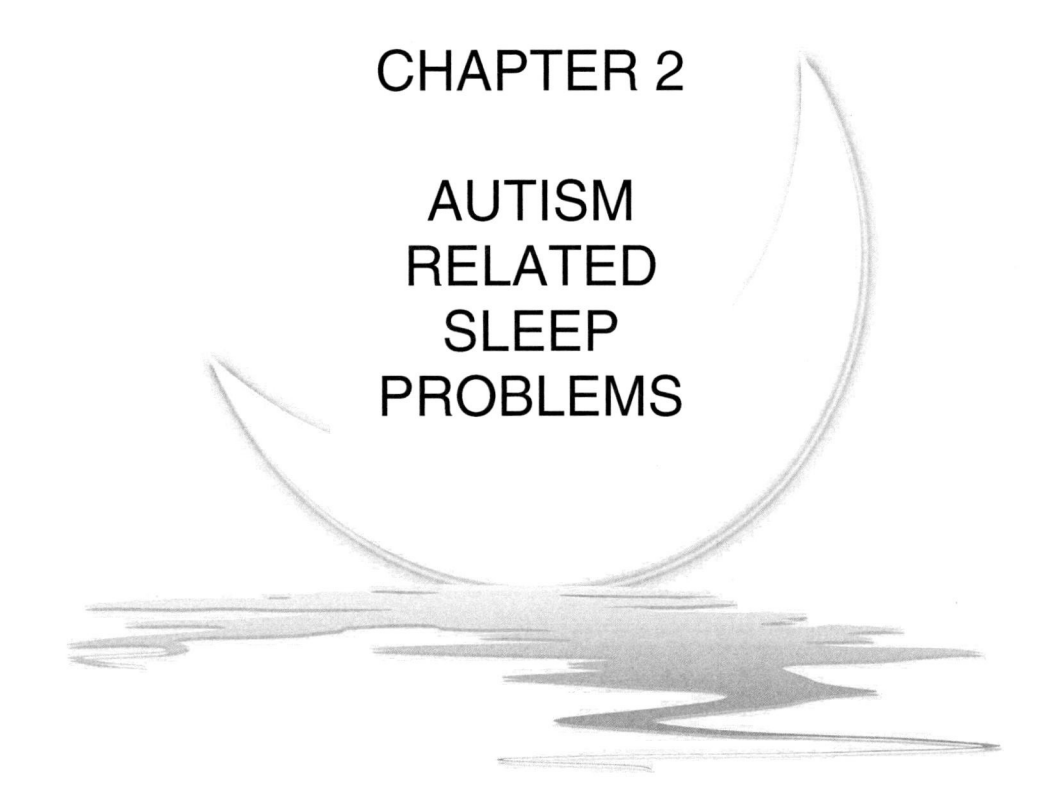

CHAPTER 2

AUTISM RELATED SLEEP PROBLEMS

COMMON SLEEP PROBLEMS ASSOCIATED WITH AUTISM...

Temporary sleep difficulties are typical. However, 40%--up to 80% of children with Autism Spectrum Disorder can have ongoing significant sleep problems with:

- *Circadian Rhythms*—The natural wake/ sleep cycles
- *Abnormal regulation*/levels of *Melatonin*, a hormone that regulates the wake/sleep cycle
- *Anxiety* about bedtime routine and social cue signals
- *Oversensitivity* to light, touch and/or sounds

WHAT SLEEP PROBLEMS OCCUR MORE OFTEN FOR PERSONS WITH AUTISM?

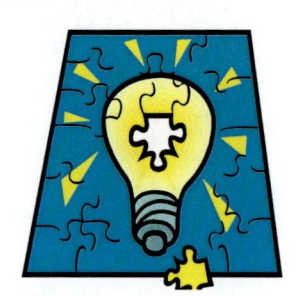

❖ *Difficulty falling asleep*

❖ *Inconsistent sleep routines**

❖ *Restlessness* or poor sleep quality

❖ *Waking early* due to lower levels of *Melatonin*** at night or hypersensitivity to sounds/light

❖ *Daytime sleepiness* due to higher levels of *Melatonin*** during the day

❖ *Nocturia* or increased need to urinate at night with increased frequency of bedwetting

❖ *Difficulty staying in bed* *or in room* due to sensory hypersensitivities, over-responsiveness or difficulty with self-regulation for calming self

* *Daytime naps typically and developmentally stop between 2 and 5 years of age.*

** *Made by body's amino acid, Tryptophan*

WHAT EFFECTS DO THESE SLEEP PROBLEMS HAVE?

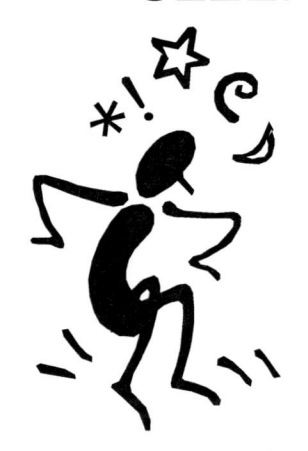

- Irritability
- Aggression
- Depression
- Hyperactivity

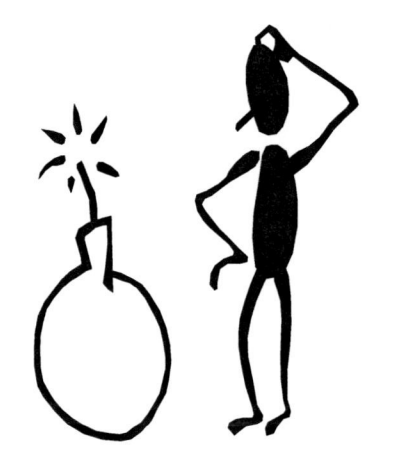

- Increased Behavioral/Socialization Problems
- Difficulty with Sustained or Focused Attention
- Poor Learning and Cognitive Performance

Parents of children with Autism Spectrum Disorder or special needs, in general, have poorer quality of sleep, sleep less, and wake earlier than typical parents.

Note: When children do not sleep, parents then do not sleep, especially if they have sensory processing needs of their own.

CHAPTER 3

HOW TO CREATE A CONDUCIVE ENVIRONMENT & FACILITATE SLEEP

AUTISM SLEEPS

TO FACILITATE HEALTHY SLEEP

To facilitate healthy sleep in a child, adolescent or adult, ask yourself…

1. ***DO YOU KEEP TO A SCHEDULE?*** Provide a routine for consistency and regularity to help the body program itself into a pattern of behavior to get "sleepy".

- For an adult it is critical to keep to a consistent bedtime daily.
- For an adolescent it is important to teach them to keep track of their activities through routine use of an agenda to get chores and homework done early enough to allow for adequate sleep time.
- For a child it is critical to keep to a routine for them to trust and rely on their caregivers through the consistency that a routine offers.
- For a special needs child, the use of a picture schedule with or without words may be needed, depending on the learning method.

2. ***IS YOUR HOME HEALTHY?*** Create a conducive environment to allow the body and mind to relax, unwind and calm to welcome the need for sleep. In order to experience healthy sleep, it is very important to develop a healthy home environment to enable this to occur. To have a healthy or "wellness" home, the use of organic or natural products is essential. These would include the areas of:

TO FACILITATE HEALTHY SLEEP
(Continued)—

 **ater** Our bodies, including our brains, are made of tissues that require a large amount of water to work. The more alkaline the water, the better our systems can function with proper hydration. Tap water can contain toxic elements that include chlorine, lead, arsenic and other impurities that increase the acidity levels. A good water system produces a highly alkaline water with a pH range of 8.5-9.5. It consists of: a multiple filtration system; minerals, including calcium; and magnetic technology that ionizes and conditions without adding salt or other chemicals.

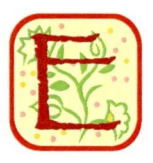 **nergy** Magnetic energy is a fundamental part of the universe. Earth itself is a giant magnet, with negative and positive (North and South) poles. Over the past few centuries, our civilization has developed structures and machines that have disrupted the flow of this energy that surrounds us. Products with magnetic technology seek to counterbalance this interruption of energy flow.

 **ight** Sunlight contains a full spectrum of light that is good for us both physically and mentally. Fluorescent lights emit only part of this spectrum and have been studied and shown to increase depression in children. Use of a full spectrum lamp recreates sunshine indoors, free of harmful rays, that can help our mood as well as our sleep/wake cycles.

 **ungs** The air we breathe is critical to allow oxygen to enter our brain and enable us to be more alert and focused to think more clearly. A proper air purifier produces laboratory-quality air consisting of an ULPA filtration system that purifies 99.999% of impurities better than HEPA filters; a patented system that produces negative ions that is like breathing ocean or mountain air; and patented technology that does not produce ozone, a toxic gas that is emitted from other systems.

TO FACILITATE HEALTHY SLEEP
(Continued)—

 **utrition** "We are what we eat" is a phrase commonly heard by many of us. The best way to take care of your nutritional needs is the natural way with wholesome foods that are developed to fill in the gaps in our diets. Whole foods provide optimum nutrition, convenience to balance busy lifestyles, and targeted nutrition for specific needs. Product benefits include mental clarity, joint and bone health, immune boosters, intestinal balance, and lowering of high cholesterol, blood pressure and blood sugar.

 **ducation** Ignorance may be bliss for some, but when it comes to our health, it can be dangerously costly in terms of illness and disease. Studies, books, online resources and other media on health and wellness are available to guide how we manage the health of our home/work environments, our family, and our own mind and bodies. It is very important that we educate ourselves on how to improve the world in which we live by implementing more organic, holistic and naturally healthy options to improve our lives and those of our loved ones.

 **kin** Keep your skin healthy by hydrating and using organic products that are botanically based, pH-corrected, cruelty-free (never tested on animals), pesticide-free, packaged in recyclable materials, and environmentally friendly. Be sure the products contain no petroleum or mineral oil, no synthetic detergents or perfumes, no artificial colors or parabens, no polyethylene glycol, and only cold-pressed oils.

 **leep** Getting the best possible sleep is important for everyone. Sleep quality has already been shown to affect virtually every other aspect of health. A good sleep system helps a person feel ready for sleep; minimizes localized pressure areas; regulates body temperature; and helps to sleep better, deeper and longer with less snoring through advanced scientific technology.

TO FACILITATE HEALTHY SLEEP
(Continued)—

The following section will provide a list of sensory strategies and suggestions that can both create a conducive and calm, relaxed environment for comfort and soothing, as well as to facilitate the body to experience healthy sleep for deeper relaxation. Since sleep is the period of time that our bodies process and integrate what was learned during the day, as well as to recover physically from our daily stresses, it is critical that we enable ourselves to benefit from the effects of deep, healing sleep. Part of this is to:

- Prepare for bedtime at dinner time.
- Keep a consistent bedtime schedule.
- Utilize products that develop a "wellness" or healthy home environment.
- Be aware of family dynamics and the tension or struggles that can interrupt the ability to be calm in a bedroom.
- Make the bedroom a serene, relaxing, warm and comfortable area that attracts the person to lie down to welcome the need for sleep time.

WHAT CAN BE DONE TO FACILITATE HEALTHY SLEEP?

AVOID...

1. **Stimulants**, such as bright or loud room colors (reds, yellows or white) and foods such as caffeine & sugar (especially carbonated sodas) at least 4-6 hours before bed.

2. **Stimulating activities** 1-2 hours before bedtime [e.g.-exercise, running, jumping, rough play, TV shows, loud/fast music, etc.].

3. **Electronics**-Keep 5 ft. or more away; images linger [television, computer & other screens].

4. **Sensory distractions** at night in/outside room.

5. **Heavy meals** 2 or more hours before bedtime; do not be stuffed or starved before going to sleep. [Begin planning for sleep at dinner time.]

WHAT CAN BE DONE TO FACILITATE HEALTHY SLEEP?

AVOID...

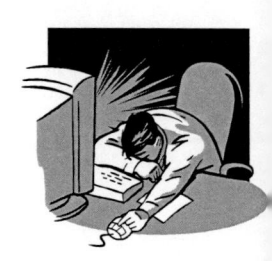

6. ***Over or Under Dressing*** depending on room temperature.

7. ***Frequent interruptions*** to the bedtime routine.

8. ***Lying down with your child*** as a regular part of your bedtime routine or using the bedroom as a "time out" area for punishment.

9. ***Picking up your child*** if he or she continues to call or fights going to sleep. Reassure him or her that you are nearby.

10. ***Quieting crying*** with food, a bottle or drink in bed...could stimulate awakening or bedwetting, create poor oral hygiene, promote tooth decay and affect bite formation.

NOTE: Check with a dentist about this and the prolonged use of a pacifier.

WHAT CAN BE DONE TO FACILITATE HEALTHY SLEEP?

DO...

1. Provide a *calming environment* with soothing wall colors (blues, greens, purples, browns or grays in pale, dark or subtle tones).
2. Establish a *consistent nighttime routine*.
3. Help provide *relaxation before bedtime*.
4. Lower *bedroom temperature* (65-62 degrees) [Keep feet warm to avoid awakening].
5. Prevent *sensory distractions* at night.
6. Keep a *sleep diary* to track time of sleep and the number of nighttime awakenings.
7. Ask Physician about *natural alternatives*.
8. Provide Preparatory, Functional & Transitional *sensory strategies* for conducive environment.

WHAT CAN BE DONE TO FACILITATE HEALTHY SLEEP? DO...

9. *Watch for signs of being OVERTIRED:*

- Rubbing or red-rimmed eyes

- Rubbing or pulling ears (if no ear concerns)

- Scratching or rubbing nose

- Rubbing face into your shoulder, blanket, etc.

- Yawning and/or arching back

10. *Schedule daily NAP times for:*

- Newborns (0-3 mos.) 4 or 5 per day, 1-3 hours

- Infants (3-6 mos.) 3 per day, 1-3 hours

- Infants (6-14 mos.) 2 per day, 1-3 hours

- Toddlers (15 mos.-3 yrs.) 1 for 2-3 hours

A CHILD'S TYPICAL BEDTIME ROUTINE

1. Have a ***light snack*** 1 hour before bath time.

2. Take a ***bath—warm water*** to calm muscles.

3. Put on ***pajamas***—especially keep feet warm; snug is relaxing for some, loose for others.

4. ***Brush teeth*** —with warm/tepid water to rinse and go to ***bathroom/potty***.

5. Make sure ***room is quiet*** and at a comfortable temperature— ***better cooler*** than warmer.

6. Read/ look at or listen to a ***book or music in the "womb" area enclosure***.

7. ***"Unwind" 30 minutes before*** going to bed.

8. Say ***good night and leave***, being sure child appears to feel safe and secure.

WHEN SHOULD SENSORY STRATEGIES BE USED?

BEDTIME PHASE 1—*PREPARATORY:*

To prepare or get ready to get into bed

BEDTIME PHASE 2—*FUNCTIONAL:*

In-bed strategies that are calming or relaxing to induce and attain a state of healthy NREM sleep

BEDTIME PHASE 3—*TRANSITIONAL:*

Strategies upon gentle awakening to prepare to begin a new day

NOTE: As with any sensory input whether external or intraoral, ***precautions and/or contraindications*** should be thoroughly considered prior to application of sensory strategies. This would include awareness of any significant medical concerns and/or hypersensitivities (e.g.—allergies, seizures, tactile defensiveness, etc.). Be aware that sensory overload could occur that could cause paleness, sweating, palpitations or agitation, as well as a nervous system "shut down" with listlessness or non-responsiveness.

WHAT TYPE OF SENSORY STRATEGIES SHOULD BE USED TO INDUCE SLEEP?

2 GENERAL TYPES OF SENSORY INPUT:

1. **EXTEROCEPTIVE [External]**

Auditory	Olfactory
Oral	Visual

   Tactile /Proprioceptive

   Vestibular

2. **INTEROCEPTIVE [Internal]**

   "GUT" FEELINGS:

Calmness	Comfort
Contentment	Happiness
Safety	Security

   Warmth

EXTEROCEPTIVE SENSORY STRATEGIES:

AUDITORY— Hearing/Sounds/Noises

1. Give a *10-minute warning* before it is time to get ready for bed. Use a timer-reinforced verbal prompt.
2. Have a *quiet period* just before bedtime.
3. Play *soothing music* or nature sounds, soft classical, instrumentals, metronome, etc.
4. Provide *white noise* to "cover" outside sounds.
5. *Speak quietly*, softly & teach *relaxation* techniques.
6. Provide *graduated music* to arouse/awaken.
7. Teach Relaxation by Reading: *The Floppy Sleep Game Book.*
8. *Whitenoiseplayer.com* for use on room computer if in room to play ocean, sleep & nature sounds, fan & other indoor sounds.
9. *Webmetronome.com* or electronic metronome.
10. Sing *soothing songs* to relax to sleep.

EXTEROCEPTIVE SENSORY STRATEGIES:

AUDITORY— (Continued)

Books-Recorded	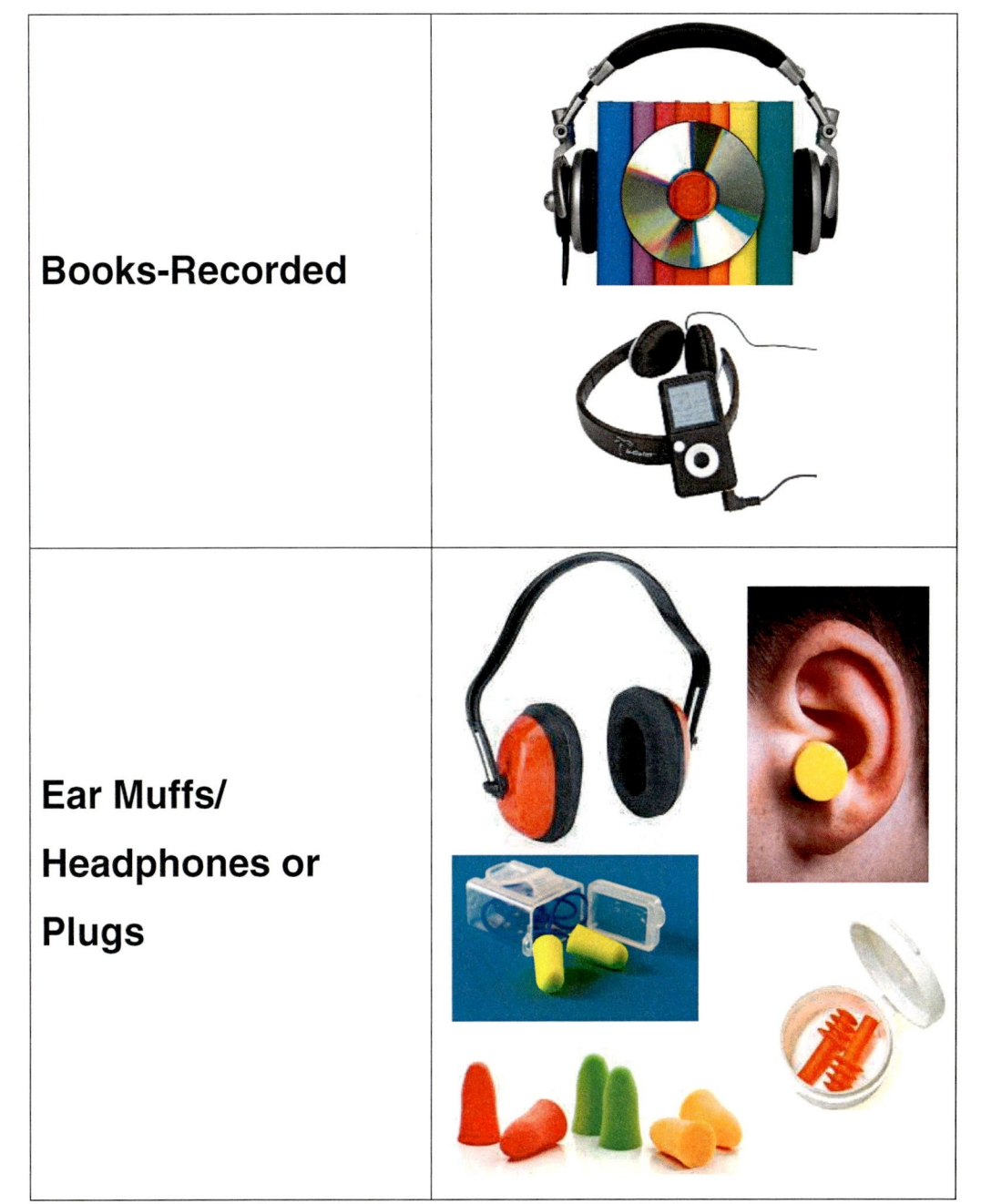
Ear Muffs/ Headphones or Plugs	

EXTEROCEPTIVE SENSORY STRATEGIES:

AUDITORY— (Continued)

Metronome: Electronic or mechanical at < 60 beats per minute	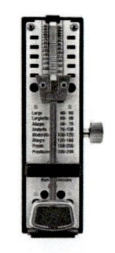 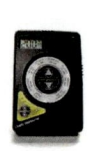 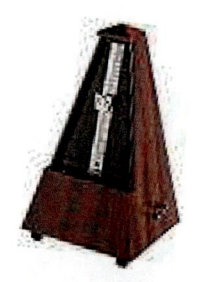
Music: Soothing, slow, rhythmic, repetitive, classical or children's songs	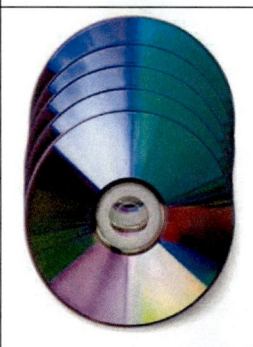 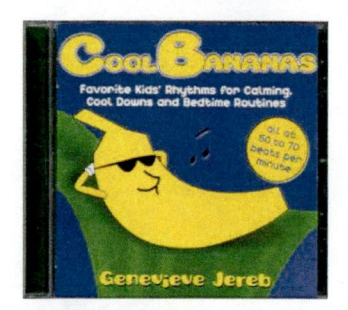 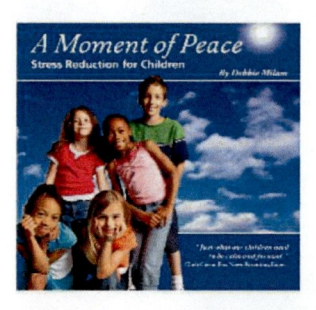
Sound Machines: White noise, nature sounds, stuffed animals with recorded heartbeat, etc.	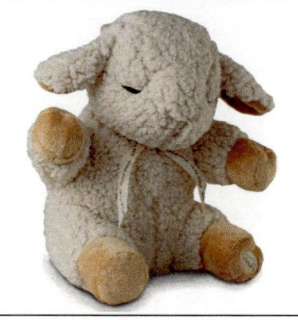 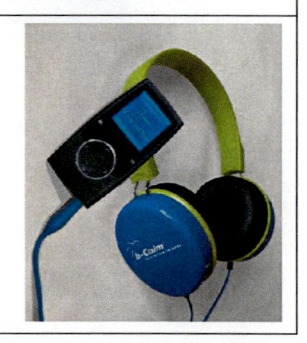

EXTEROCEPTIVE SENSORY STRATEGIES:

AUDITORY— (Continued)

Timers: Digital, electronic, mechanical, sand or visual	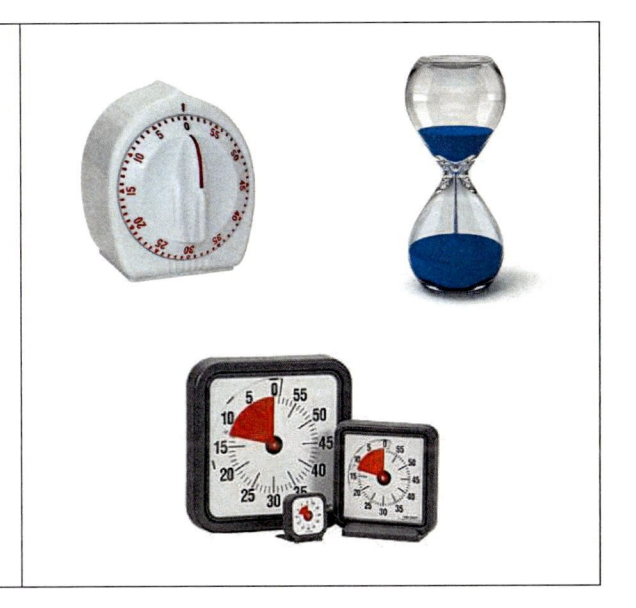

EXTEROCEPTIVE SENSORY STRATEGIES:

OLFACTORY— Smell or Breathe

1. Apply *AROMATHERAPY* formulas as needed:

   A. <u>Aromatic Massage Oil to Calm</u>—

   (A relaxing hand or foot massage blend)

   2 Tablespoons warm vegetable oil

   5-10 drops essential oil of Lavender & Mandarin

   DIRECTIONS: Mix together; massage feet/hands

   towards heart with firm, gentle pressure.

EXTEROCEPTIVE SENSORY STRATEGIES:

OLFACTORY— Smell or Breathe (Continued)

1. Apply *AROMATHERAPY* formulas as needed:

    B. <u>Room Spray to Relax</u>—

    1 Cup distilled or filtered water

    20 drops Mandarin, 10 drops Lavender, 5 drops
    Marjoram & 5 drops Sandalwood essential oils

    DIRECTIONS: Place above in spray bottle with fine
    mist nozzle in above order; shake well before each
    spray; mist room, furniture, pillowcase/bedding, etc.

    C. <u>Room Diffuser Synergy Blend for Overactivity</u>—

    4 parts Lavender essential oil

    1 part each Clary Sage, Cedarwood & Sandalwood
    essential oils

    DIRECTIONS: Use for *inhalation only*. Use
    teaspoon of each in diffuser. Diffuse 15 minutes
    before bedtime.

    Essences will last several hours. Use up to 3 times
    per day---DO NOT OVERUSE!

EXTEROCEPTIVE SENSORY STRATEGIES:

OLFACTORY— Smell or Breathe (Continued)

2. Use an *AIR PURIFIER* that ionizes the air with a negative charge via negative-ion generation to provide forest-air freshness, the exhilarating feeling produced by high levels of negative ions in natural settings without the production of toxic ozone.

3. Use CANDLES with scents that are relaxing, such as Lavender, Vanilla, etc.

4. Personal, nasal inhalers also tend to calm, and help open air passageways as do other over-the-counter ointments that could be recommended by a physician or pharmacist.

Air Purifier: Production of clean air with negative ions for greater breathing ease	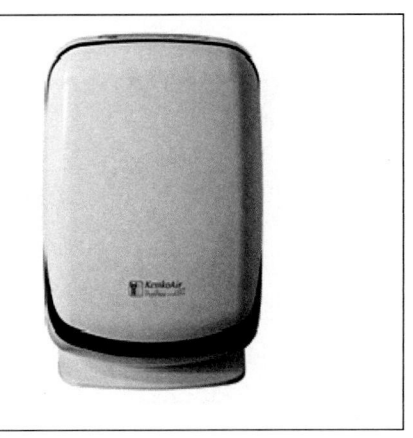

EXTEROCEPTIVE SENSORY STRATEGIES:

OLFACTORY— Smell or Breathe (Continued)

Aromatherapy-Diffusers: Battery-Powered, Candle Heated, Electrical, Plug-In or Room-Sized, Vaporizer with Lighted Diffuser Or Reed Diffuser	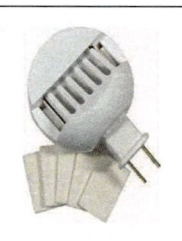 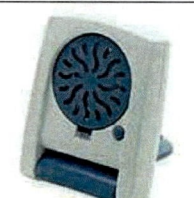 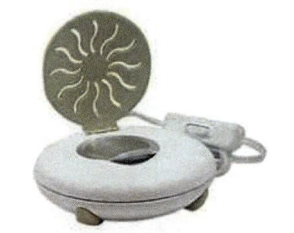 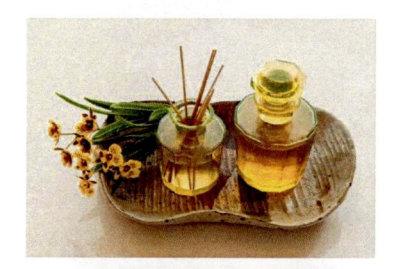
Candles-Scented	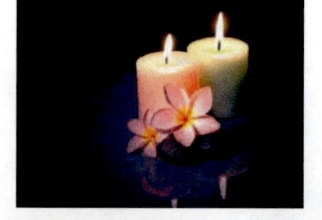
Inhalers: Personal	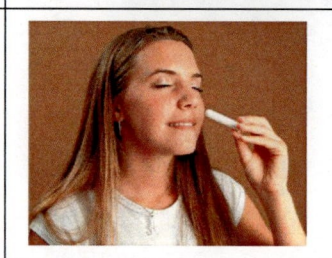 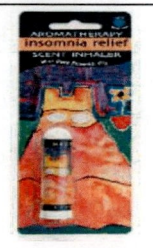

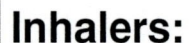

EXTEROCEPTIVE SENSORY STRATEGIES:
ORAL—Taste or Chewing/Sucking Need

1. Before bedtime *light snack high in Tryptophan,* the sleep-inducing amino acid/hormone, such as warm milk, cottage cheese, yogurt, pineapples, plums, bananas, eggs, turkey, sesame seeds, cashews, peanuts.

2. Combine above with *complex carbohydrates* like whole grain cereals, bread or potatoes. [Examples: Peanut butter sandwich with ground sesame seeds, whole grain cereal or oatmeal with milk, oatmeal cookies with warm milk]

3. Provide an *oral "tool"* for child to suck or chew to calm down as needed.

4. Have a *drink of filtered, mineralized and ionized water and/or juice* at bedside to end and also begin the day with brain/body hydration.

EXTEROCEPTIVE SENSORY STRATEGIES:

ORAL—Taste or Chewing/Sucking Need (Continued)

5. Be sure breakfast contains *simple carbohydrates* for energy *& protein* for brain food, with adequate hydration to recharge body's tissues.

NOTE: 5 FOODS FOR DEEP SLEEP

Per Dr. Pina LoGiudice, ND, the following foods should be eaten ½-1 hour before bedtime:

- **Pumpkin Seed Powder** mixed with carbohydrates (applesauce)—very high in Tryptophan;
- **Tart Cherries**—high in Melatonin (juice is 10 times the strength of fresh, but higher in sugar);
- **PULQUE,** an alcoholic drink from Mexico made from agave plant—very high in Tryptophan;

EXTEROCEPTIVE SENSORY STRATEGIES:

ORAL—Taste or Chewing/Sucking Need (Continued)

- *Scottish Oatmeal*, a Nervine high in Tryptophan and Melatonin that reduces Serotonin levels for increased alertness: ¼ cup for children; ½ cup for adolescents and adults;
- *Dandelion Greens* that help the liver process foods (cook like collards for dinner).

Cheeses: Cottage or other types of natural cheeses contain Tryptophan which induces sleep	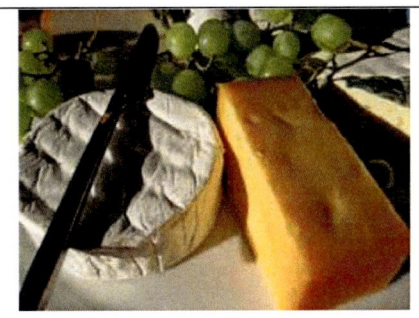
Chewies: Pacifier for infants, teething rings or dental sticks, assorted chewy tubes or forms	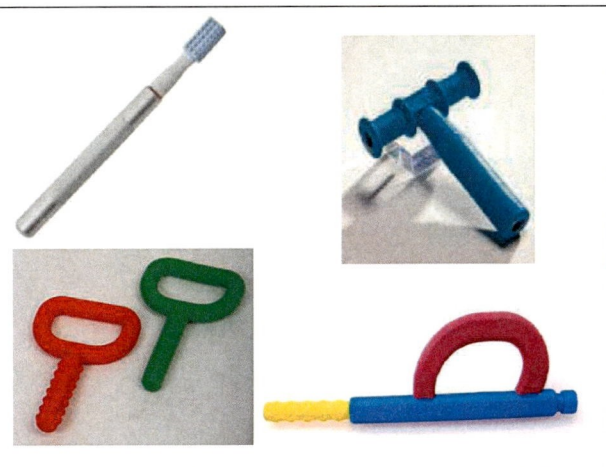

NOTE: A dentist or orthodontist should be consulted for prolonged use of any oral appliance.

EXTEROCEPTIVE SENSORY STRATEGIES:

ORAL—Taste or Chewing/Sucking Need (Continued)

Fruits: Bananas, Pineapples, Plums or Tart Cherries (Fresh or Juice)-8 oz. 2 hours before bed & in morning to reset internal clock thru increased Melatonin when taken at regularly scheduled times	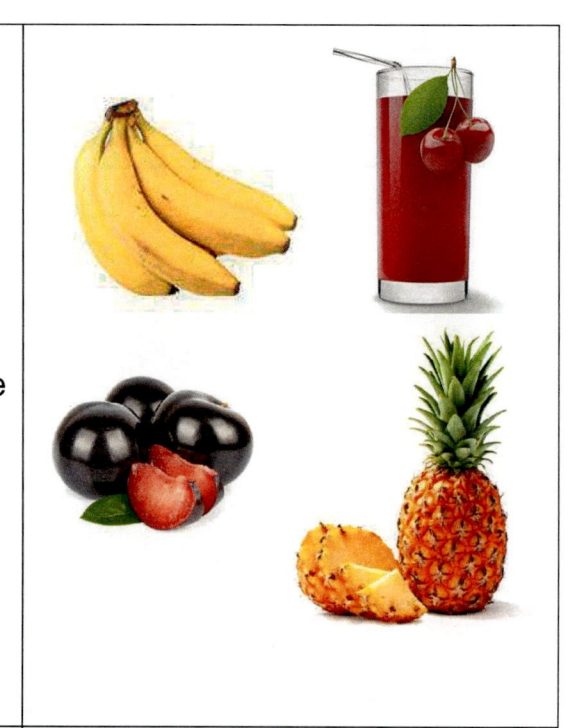
Honey: Pure, raw honey is best to reduce OREXIN (a neurotransmitter) that increases alertness.	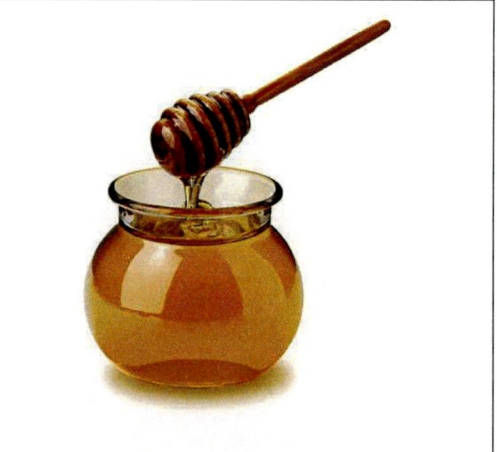

NOTE: Consult a pediatrician for age when a child can safely intake honey.

EXTEROCEPTIVE SENSORY STRATEGIES:

ORAL—Taste or Chewing/Sucking Need (Continued)

Magnesium Rich Foods: (↓ Sweating) Almonds, Bananas, Basil, Broccoli, Barley, Black Beans, Brazil Nuts, Buckwheat Flour, Cacao (Semisweet Chocolate), Chives, Cornmeal, Dill, Flax Seeds, Halibut, Oat Bran, Okra, Pine Nuts, Pumpkin/Squash Seeds, Soybeans, Spearmint, Spinach, Sunflower Seeds, Watermelon Seeds, White Beans, Whole Wheat Flour

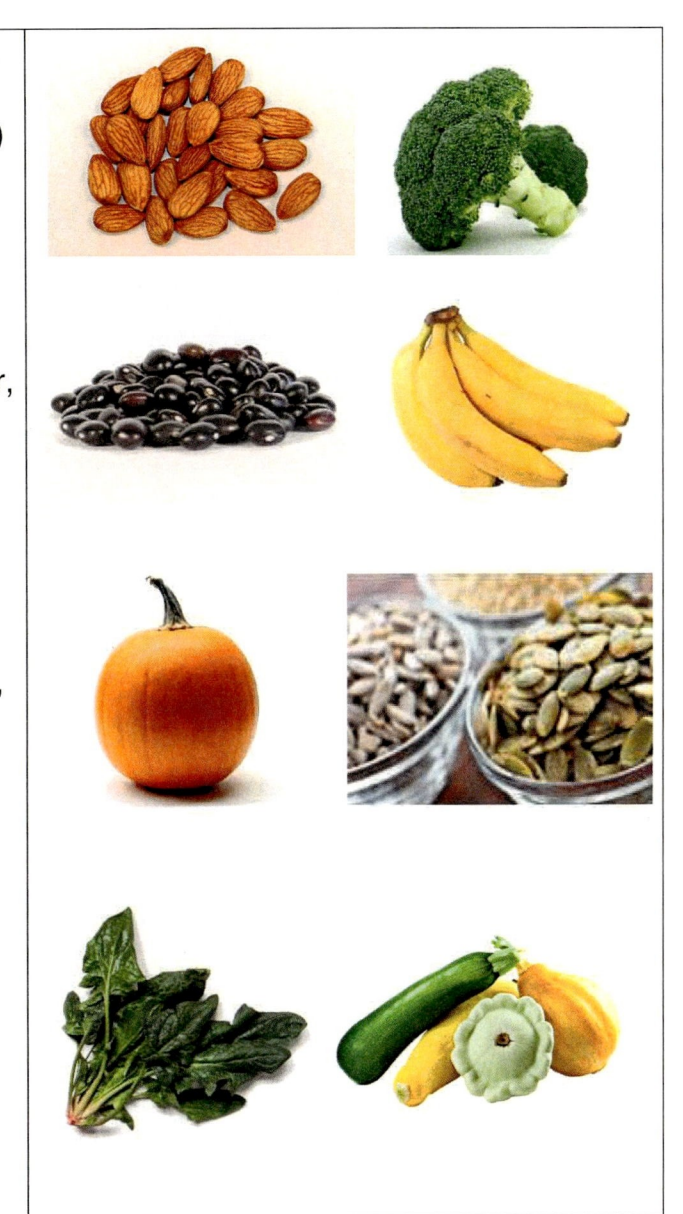

EXTEROCEPTIVE SENSORY STRATEGIES:

ORAL—Taste or Chewing/Sucking Need (Continued)

Milk: Room temperature or warm [e.g.-oatmeal or peanut butter cookie]	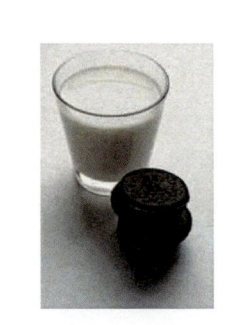 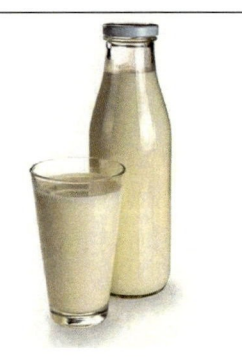
Non-Alcoholic Beer (Malt, Hops) To increase GABA production, a brain tranquilizer	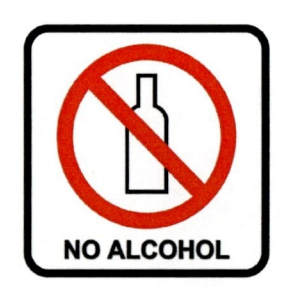 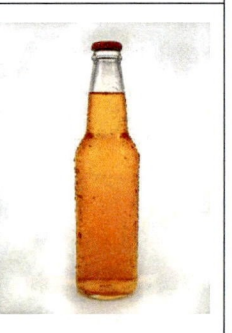
Oatmeal: Irish or Scottish (preferable) or other steel cut versus rolled oats with low/ no sugar or honey. Irish oatmeal is chewier and nuttier in flavor than other types of oatmeal. Because Irish or Scottish Oatmeal is less processed than rolled	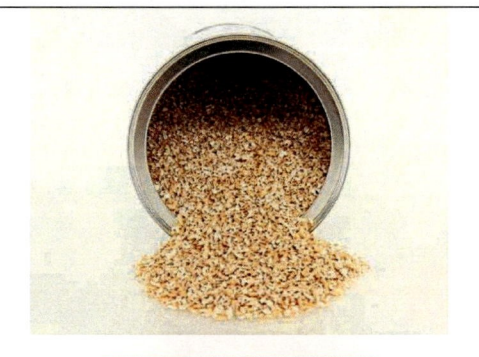 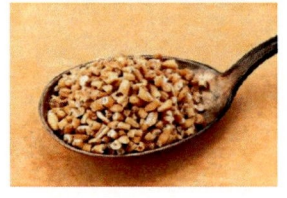

EXTEROCEPTIVE SENSORY STRATEGIES:

ORAL—Taste or Chewing/Sucking Need (Continued)

Oatmeal: oats or instant oatmeal, it is higher in fiber, B vitamins, calcium and protein. There is some evidence that oatmeal can help lower cholesterol levels.	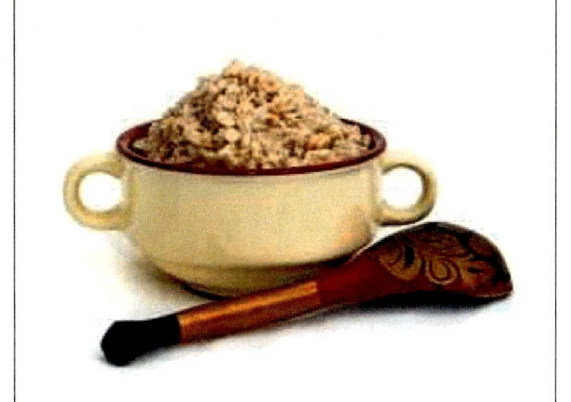
Popcorn: Light; sprinkled with Parmesan cheese	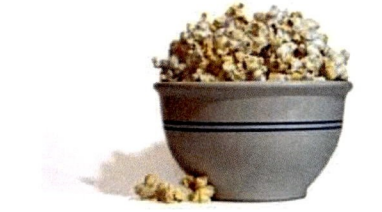
Protein: Black Bean, Eggs, Turkey, Veggie Whey, Zucchini or other patty	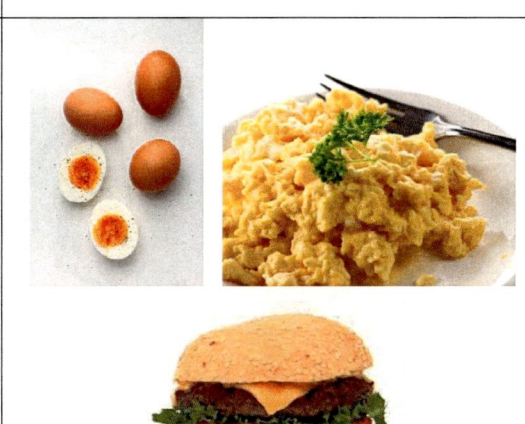

EXTEROCEPTIVE SENSORY STRATEGIES:

ORAL—Taste or Chewing/Sucking Need (Continued)

Pudding: Homemade without preservatives is best.	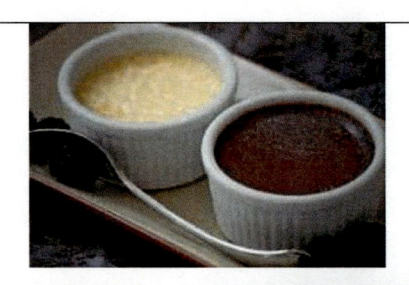
Seeds: (Increase Tryptophan & help manage stress/ anxiety) Chia (2 oz.), Cumin, Sesame, Sunflower seeds or Peanuts/ Peanut Butter	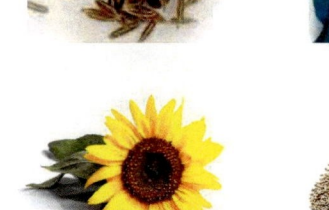 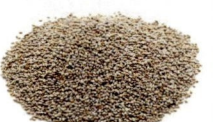 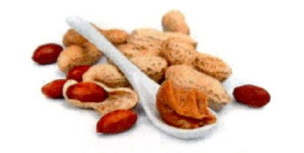
Spices: Cinnamon, Nutmeg or Vanilla	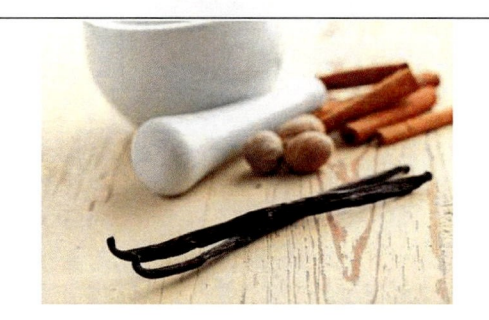

EXTEROCEPTIVE SENSORY STRATEGIES:

ORAL—Taste or Chewing/Sucking Need (Continued)

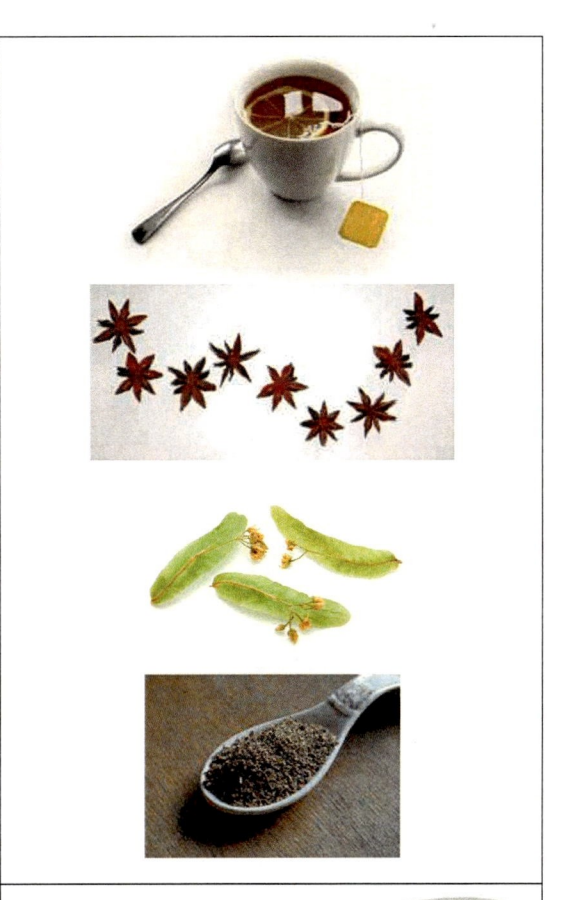

Teas:

(Digestive Aids that reduce

stomach gas &/or calm)

Anise (Star) Seeds,

Chamomile (Flower),

Tilia (Linden Flower Leaves)

or

Valerian (Root)

Water:

(Alkaline-best/preferable)

Filtered,

Mineralized

& Ionized

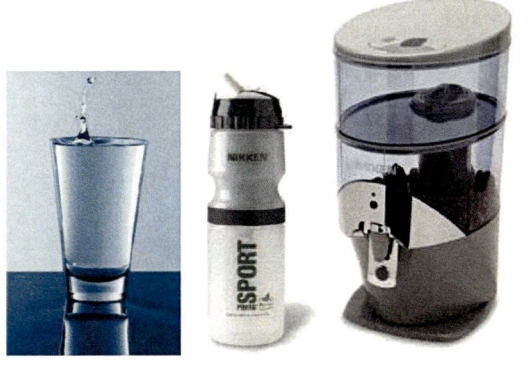

EXTEROCEPTIVE SENSORY STRATEGIES:

ORAL—Taste or Chewing/Sucking Need (Continued)

Wheat Germ: (1 tsp.) To decrease stress/ anxiety with Vitamin B_6; preferably whole grain	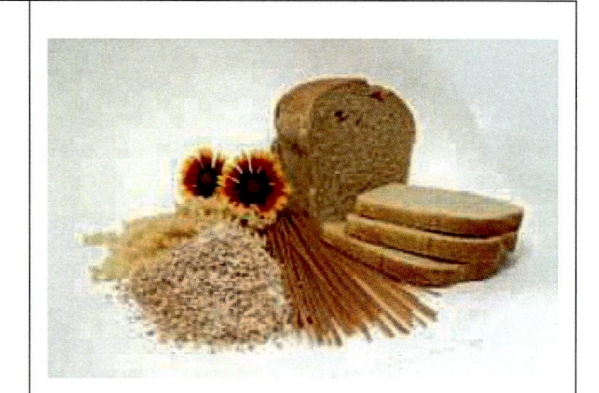
Yogurt: Plain or Vanilla with natural fruit or honey is preferred.	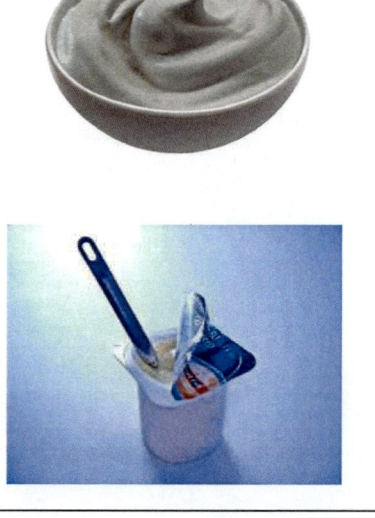

Note: A combination of above ingredients is even more effective than using them singularly [e.g. peanut butter on a wheat cracker with a glass of vanilla milk warmed with a stick of cinnamon, yogurt with fresh cherries or pineapple chunks, etc.].

EXTEROCEPTIVE SENSORY STRATEGIES:

TACTILE (Touch) /PROPRIOCEPTIVE (Joint Position Sense)—

1. *SELECT A BED OR SLEEP SYSTEM* that best suits the sensory system & that most invites you &/or your child to sleep. Selections include:

- Standard coiled mattress and box springs
- Multiple/heavy comforters or sleeping bags
- An inflatable air or water mattress
- Memory or "T" foam mattress
- Magnetic sleep system*

   NOTE: The use of magnetic products is contraindicated and should be kept at a safe distance from individuals with Vagal Nerve Stimulators (VNS), Pacemakers, Insulin pumps, shunts and/or metal implants made of materials that are attracted to magnets. The individual's physician should be contacted to determine what would be deemed as a "safe" distance.

2. *PROVIDE POSITIONING AIDS* to support posture & comfort.

EXTEROCEPTIVE SENSORY STRATEGIES:

TACTILE (Touch) /PROPRIOCEPTIVE (Joint Position Sense)— (Continued)

3. *FOLLOW A BRUSHING PROGRAM* with or without joint compressions, depending on what is most calming.

4. *PROVIDE A COMFORT ITEM*, cloth, blanket or stuffed animal to hug (can be weighted, textured or with vibration).

5. PROVIDE *MASSAGE OR PERCUSSION* on back/torso to calm.

6. TRY *BRUSHING* hair *or STROKING* arms/legs.

7. Provide *HEAVY PRESSURE* to get to bed &/or in bed (weighted blanket, multiple sleeping bags, back & limb massage, joint compressions, bean bag press, etc.)

8. Use *TIGHT SHEETS OR SWADDLING* to calm.

EXTEROCEPTIVE SENSORY STRATEGIES:

TACTILE (Touch) /PROPRIOCEPTIVE (Joint Position Sense)— (Continued)

Brushing (Dry):

Back (Relax/Detoxify), Hair (Relaxation) or *Arms and Legs, [For use of a **Brushing Program*** contact a trained Occupational Therapist to implement.]

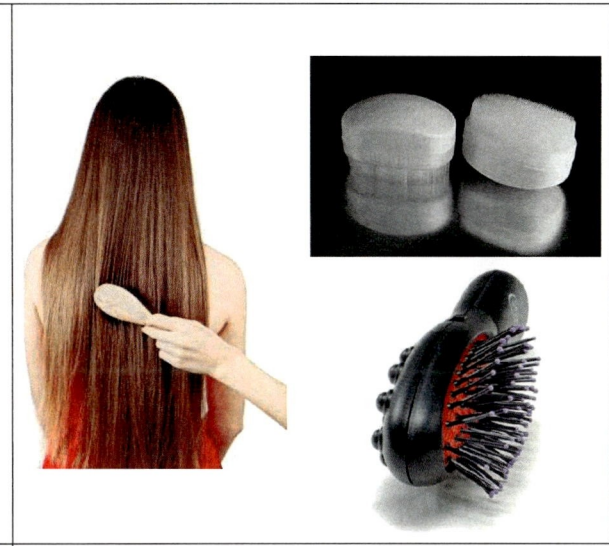

Cushions:

Positioning for comfort and/or pressure relief: **Soldier**-on back/face up; **Sleeping Beauty**-on side & most preferable or **Dead Man's Float**- on stomach, head turned & arms/stomach under pillow; Vibrating/Textured Pillows and/or Neck Cushion

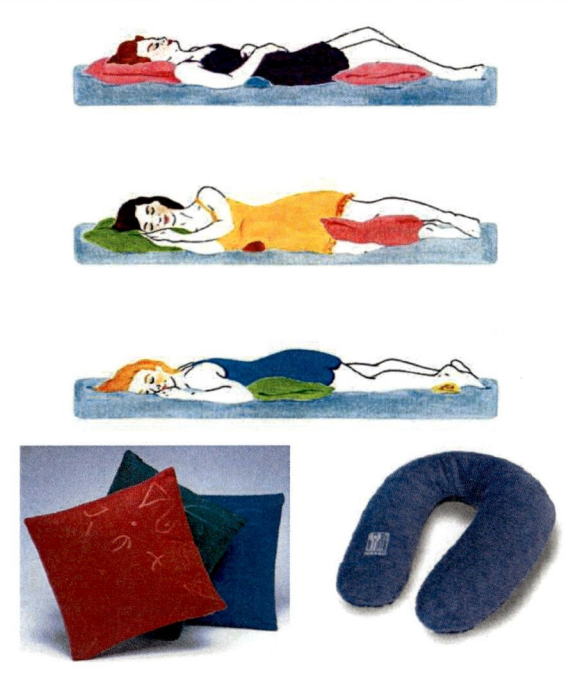

EXTEROCEPTIVE SENSORY STRATEGIES:

TACTILE (Touch) /PROPRIOCEPTIVE (Joint Position Sense)— (Continued)

Comforters: For swaddling, warmth and/or pressure	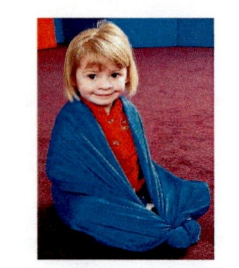 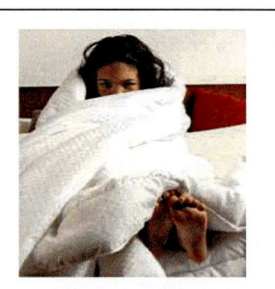
Deep Pressure/ Vibration: Using hands, balls or devices on shoulders, back, arms and/or legs	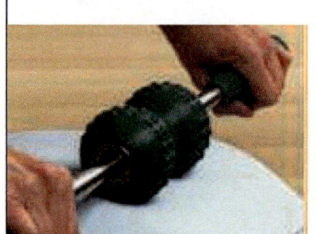 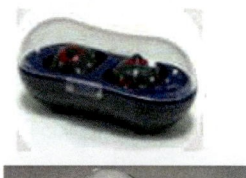
Mattress: Air, Coiled, Foam, Water or Magnetic topper	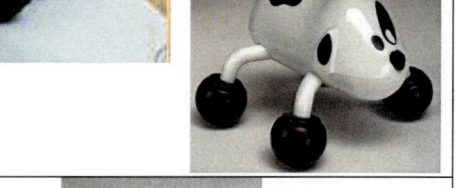 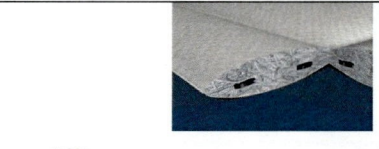
Stress Reducers: Fidgets or Squeeze balls	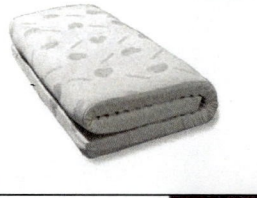 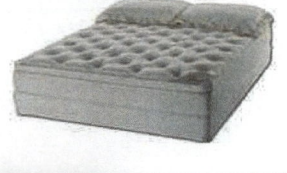 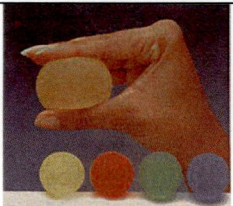

EXTEROCEPTIVE SENSORY STRATEGIES:

TACTILE (Touch) / PROPRIOCEPTIVE (Joint Position Sense)— (Continued)

Weighted Items: Blanket, Sleeping bags, "Snake", pad, etc.	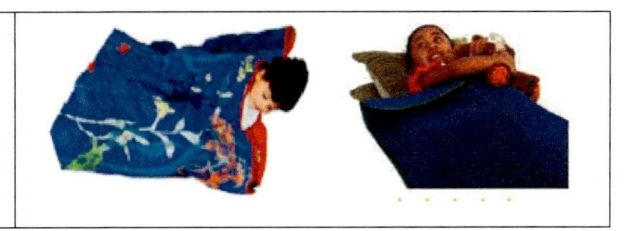

VESTIBULAR—Movement

1. *Waterbed mattress* can provide movement from full wave to waveless. The more wave action, the greater the vestibular or movement impact.

2. *Gentle rocking or rolling* in bed in side-lying position or on stomach can be very calming.

3. *Gentle swinging* in small, slow arcs can be relaxing and calming.

4. *Gliders* provide *linear movements* & calm in small increments of movement.

EXTEROCEPTIVE SENSORY STRATEGIES:

VESTIBULAR—Movement

Glider (Preferable), Swing, Upright or Floor Rocker: Gentle, slow, very even, rhythmic motion	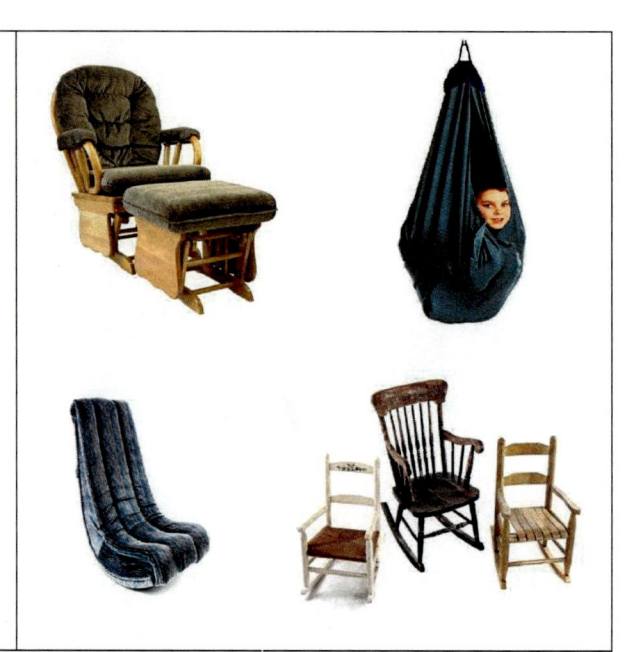

VISUAL—Sights

1. Use a *picture schedule* to teach bedtime routine.

2. Paint the walls in the bedroom in *calm tones* to relax the eyes in hues of:

   ❖ BLUE: The most tranquilizing color—It calms tension and increases feelings of well-being. When the eye sees blue, the brain releases eleven neurotransmitters that relax the body, and may result in a reduction of temperature, perspiration and appetite.

EXTEROCEPTIVE SENSORY STRATEGIES:

VISUAL—Sights (Continued)

- ❖ GREEN: Also a calming color—In response to this serene color, blood Histamine levels may rise, resulting in reduced sensitivity to food allergies. Antigens may be stimulated for overall better immune system healing.

- ❖ GRAY: The most neutral color.

- ❖ BROWN: Promotes a sense of security, relaxation, and reduces fatigue—For some it can be too dark a color to use in a room, but it can be used on an accent or "brain rest" wall.

3. Provide *warm light* (orange hues) in evening before bed to simulate sunset.

4. Provide a *"WOMB IN A ROOM"*, an enclosed area, for calming activities before going to bed.

5. Place a *soothing light* to calm (dynamic/static).

6. Add room darkening drapes/shades or provide a sleep mask to help block out light and/or thoughts

EXTEROCEPTIVE SENSORY STRATEGIES:

VISUAL—Sights (Continued)

6. that will not "turn off" in the mind.

7. Look at a *calming book* of interest.

8. Provide *gradual, bright-light (full spectrum)* therapy to awaken gently in the morning.

Books or Relaxing Pictures	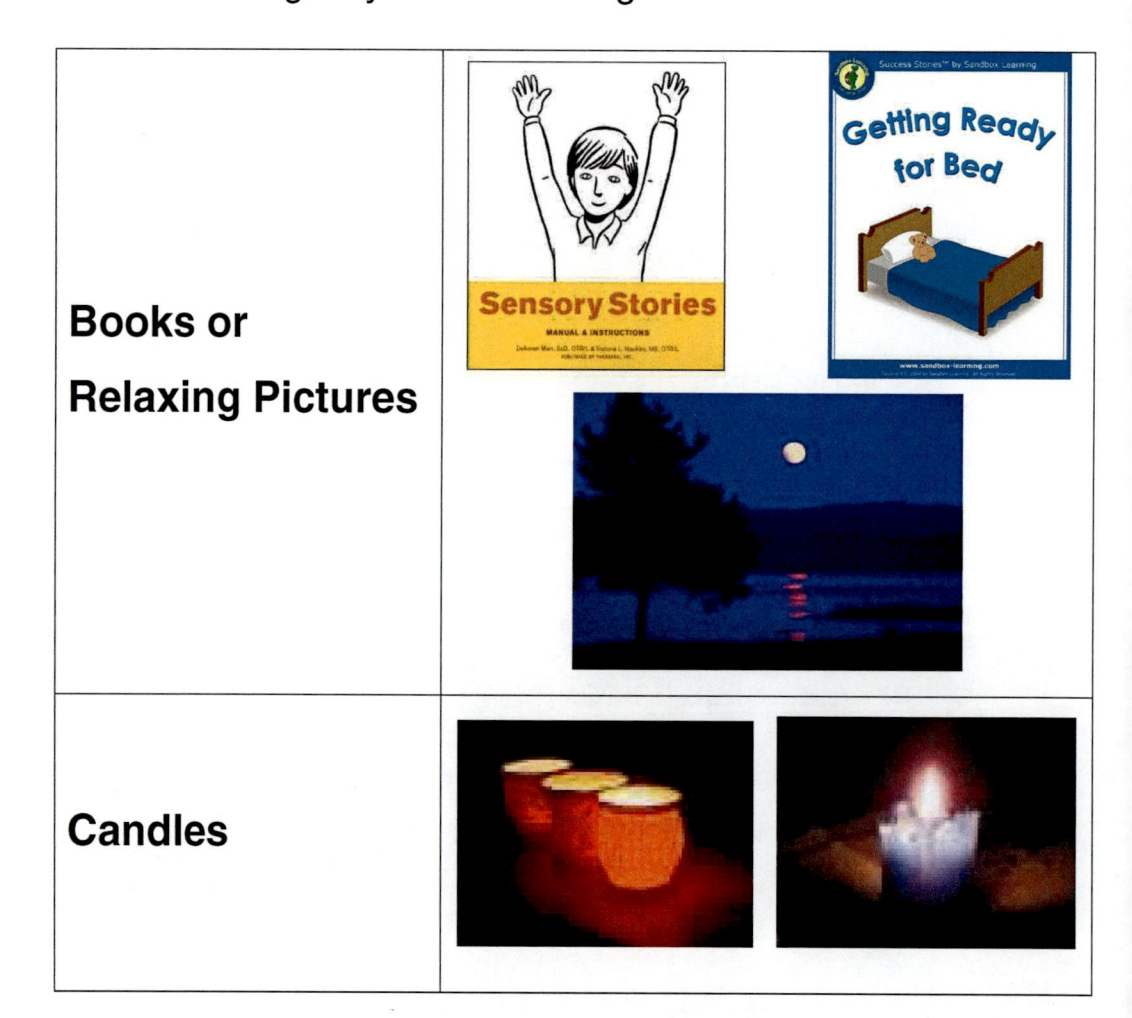
Candles	

EXTEROCEPTIVE SENSORY STRATEGIES:

VISUAL—Sights (Continued)

Full Spectrum Lighting: For graduated awakening as sunshine; helps reset biological clock with 15 minutes exposure each morning.	
Lava Lamps or Bubble Tubes	
Night Light	
Overhead or Wall Projections: Static or very slow moving stars, lights, etc.	

EXTEROCEPTIVE SENSORY STRATEGIES:

VISUAL—Sights (Continued)

Salt Rock Lamp or other lighted object with a low light, warm glow	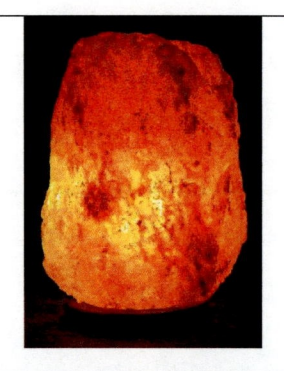
Sleep Mask: To block out light, as well as ease mental tension, and calm with far-infrared material for soothing, deep heat.	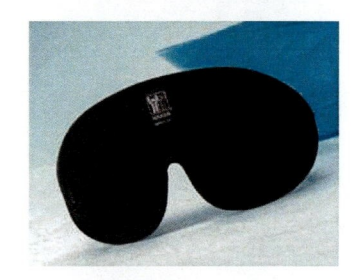
Tent: Bed type or floor type in corner to make "womb in a room"	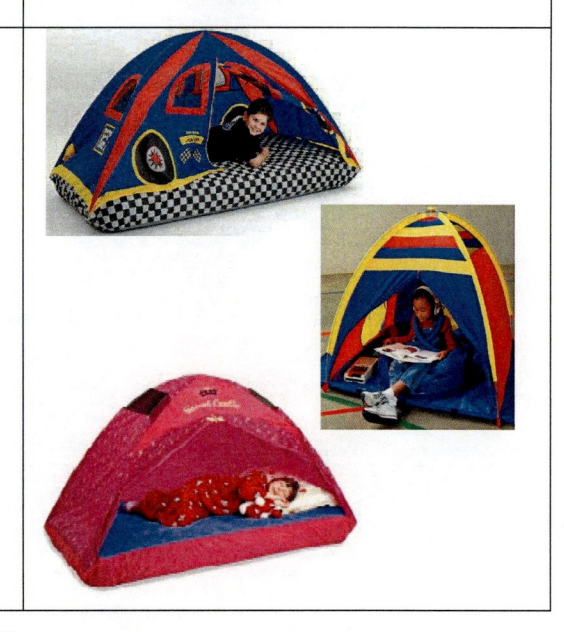

INTEROCEPTIVE SENSORY STRATEGIES:

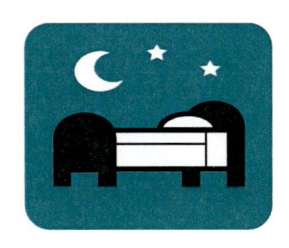

1. *Diurnal* (day/night) *patterning* is important to regulate circadian (sleep/wake) rhythms for all ages.

2. The *sleep system* used is the most important component or strategy/item to provide the comfort and relaxation needed to make bedtime a pleasurable time to anticipate.

3. Facilitating positive self-esteem is critical to the ability of the person to feel secure enough to enable a positive sleep experience.

4. Giving affection with appropriate touch to further calm and support emotionally.

5. Inducing a sense of security to help reduce anxiety, particularly for a child, would include dispelling fears of the dark, ghosts, bugs, "monsters", etc.

INTEROCEPTIVE SENSORY

STRATEGIES: (Continued)

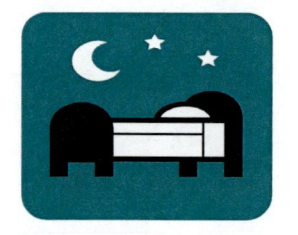

Key words to implement the above include:

- ❖ A Night Light

- ❖ Comforting Words

- ❖ Gentle or Bear Hugs

- ❖ Kisses and Soft Voice

- ❖ Listening to Talk Radio

- ❖ Review of Day's Events

- ❖ Singing Soothing Songs

- ❖ Pictures of Family or Friends

- ❖ Listening to a Recorded Voice

- ❖ Reassuring Parent(s) Is/Are Near

- ❖ Phone Call from Significant Person

- ❖ Rubbing Shoulders, Hand or Forehead

- ❖ "Monster Spray"

  [See next page for directions/recipe.]

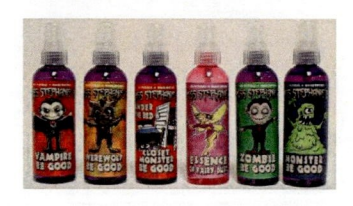

INTEROCEPTIVE SENSORY STRATEGIES:
(Continued)

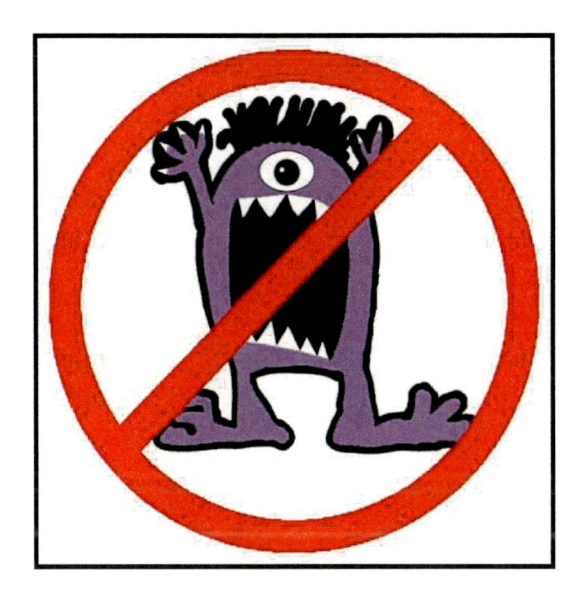

"MONSTER SPRAY"

DIRECTIONS:

1. Obtain plastic, spray bottle that is easily pushed or squeezed.

2. Fill with distilled or purified water.

3. Add drops of lavender or a calming essential oil to easily smell scent.

4. Add food coloring as desired for visually soothing effect.

5. Add above label to front of bottle if desired.

6. Spray area(s) of room where "monsters" or bugs are needed to be dispelled to reassure child.

7. <u>Recite poem</u>:
   "Monster, monster, go away! Don't come back another day!"

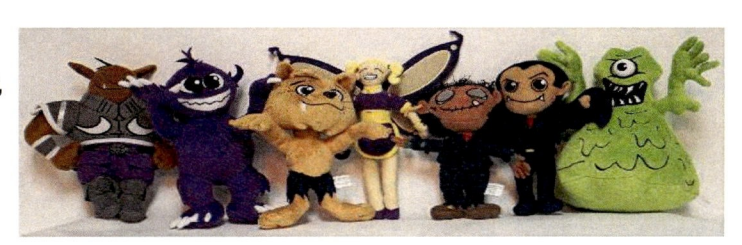

SAMPLE BEDTIME SCHEDULE

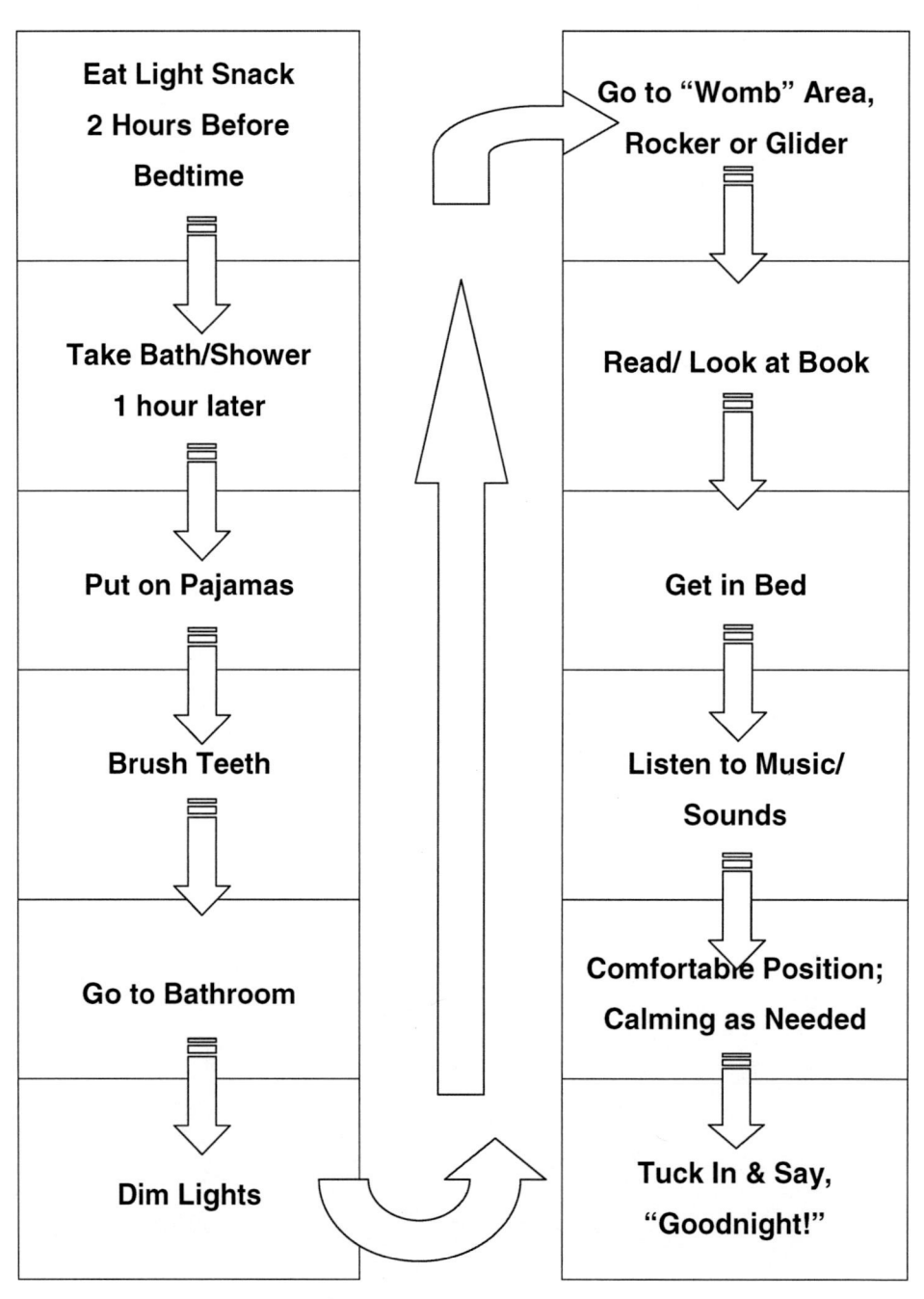

Eat Light Snack 2 Hours Before Bedtime

Take Bath/Shower 1 hour later

Put on Pajamas

Brush Teeth

Go to Bathroom

Dim Lights

Go to "Womb" Area, Rocker or Glider

Read/ Look at Book

Get in Bed

Listen to Music/ Sounds

Comfortable Position; Calming as Needed

Tuck In & Say, "Goodnight!"

CHAPTER 4

IMPLEMENTING A HEALTHY ROUTINE WITH

SENSORY SLEEP STRATEGIES

AUTISM SLEEPS

SELECTING APPROPRIATE SENSORY STRATEGIES

The key to knowing which sensory strategies to try is to identify what the activities or actions are that the person with the sleep difficulty enjoys or the behaviors that are proving to be most challenging in helping the person to slow his or her internal "clock" to allow sleep to occur. Below is a list of typical indicators that could help select the sensory strategies that would have the greatest impact on the person's sensory systems to relax and calm them enough to induce deeper sleep:

The person is observed to…	SENSORY AREA
1. Enjoy hugs or back/ neck rubs 2. Handle or touch objects often, especially with a variety of textures 3. Have shaky or "nervous" hands 4. Have difficulty or is fidgety in sitting 5. Appear to be anxious or expresses anxiety, especially in darkened rooms 6. Love to hold and/or hug animals	SKIN

SELECTING APPROPRIATE SENSORY [Continued]
STRATEGIES

The person is observed to…	SENSORY AREA
⇨ 7. Enjoy smelling objects or persons 8. Enjoy wearing cologne or perfume 9. Use or smell scented lotions 10. Have difficulty breathing through nose 11. Smell foods before eating	LUNGS
⇨ 12. Enjoy looking at pictures and/or reading books or magazines 13. Watch television or view the computer often 14. Prefer watching movies on an outing 15. Stare at lights, especially if moving 16. Have sensitivity to bright light 17. Use sunglasses or cover eyes often	EYES
⇨ 18. Enjoy and calms when listening to music or recorded books 19. Respond to soft voice when addressed 20. Covers ears often for unknown reasons 21. Appear overly sensitive to specific noises and/or loud sounds	EARS
⇨ 22. Enjoy running or physical activities 23. Prefer a physical activity as an outing 24. Be fidgety in sitting or unable to sit still for the duration of a typical activity with peers 25. Enjoy swinging or movement to calm self	POSITION

SELECTING APPROPRIATE SENSORY [Continued]
STRATEGIES

The person is observed to…	SENSORY AREA
26. Be unable to calm self except with food 27. Enjoy eating as a preferred outing 28. Be a picky eater or over-focused on eating 29. Have difficulty with food tastes / textures, especially those resistive when chewing with preference for soft or bland foods 30. Calm self or focus with sucking or chewing 31. Chew gum or other throughout the day 32. Chew on shirt or other inanimate objects	ORAL (YUMMY)

Once the appropriate area(s) is/are checked, then a list of specific sensory sleep strategies can be reviewed to note those that would pertain to the identified sensory area(s). [Review the next section.] The strategy area(s) activities can be implemented as part of the Preparatory and Functional sensory strategies to facilitate sleep. These are utilized during the sample BEDTIME ROUTINE or time schedule located after the list of sleep strategies.

SENSORY SLEEP STRATEGIES

SENSORY AREA: [Touch / Tactile Sense]

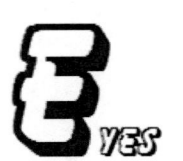

• Warm bath or shower 1 hour before bed	• Loose or snug pajamas, as tolerated, that calm and relax
• Foot rub or massage	• Back rub or massage
• Face— gentle massage	• Hair brushed or stroked
• Palm pressure at temples	• Forehead/temple rubs
• Lotion on arms &/or legs	• Cool room temperature

SENSORY AREA: [Respiration / Olfactory Sense]

• Walk or light exercise 1 hour or more before bed time for 5 minutes or less	• Aromatherapy with *essential oils* to open airways, relax and/or calm:
• Air purification system that cleans and ionizes	➢ Eucalyptus ➢ Peppermint
• Clear/open nasal passages if congested (saline spray, cool mist vaporizer, etc.)	➢ Tea Tree ➢ Cinnamon ➢ Lavender

SENSORY AREA: [Sight / Visual Sense]

• Picture schedule for routine	• ↓ Distracters (exciting, fast or stimulating items)
• Night light [warm tones]	
• Salt Rock or Lava Lamp	• Slow moving or static ceiling projection
• Read or look at a book	
• Dimmed or rope lighting	• Corner/bed tent/"womb" area

SENSORY AREA: [Hearing / Auditory Sense]

• White noise machine or fan	• Classical music [< 60 bpm]*
• Listen to a book or a CD	• Soothing music [< 60 bpm]
• Nature sounds— waterfall, ocean waves, wind, crickets, etc. (recorded or electronic)	• Metronome [< 60 bpm] * bpm = beats per minute
	• Ear plugs or headphones

SENSORY AREA: [Joints/ Proprioceptive & Movement/ Vestibular Senses]

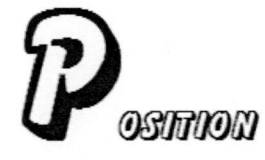

• "Womb" area— bean bag lying 30 minutes before bed	• Calming Sleep System [dense foam or magnetic pad]
• Glider rocking 30 min. prior	• Body pillow to "spoon"/hug
• Multiple sleeping bags	• Weighted blanket
• Percussion on back	• Pet or stuffed animal to hug
• Gentle rocking in bed	• Multiple bed pillows

SENSORY SLEEP STRATEGIES [Continued]

SENSORY AREA: [Eating or Drinking / Oral Sense]

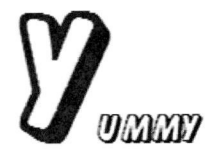

DETOXIFICATION AID:	MELATONIN RICH FOODS:

DETOXIFICATION AID:

- WATER [3 hours before bed and in morning]

TRYPTOPHAN-RICH FOODS:

- Cottage & other cheeses
- Chew Chia seeds (2 Tbsp.)
- Peanuts/Peanut butter
- Sesame seeds/butter
- Milk—Warm or tepid
- Pineapples, plums
- Turkey patty, etc.
- Sunflower seeds
- Popcorn-Light
- Oatmeal *
- Pudding
- Yogurt
- Eggs

DIGESTIVE AIDS:

- Cumin Seeds ($\downarrow$gas/ bloating and discomfort)
- Valerian Tea (sedative)
- Tilia (Tilo) Tea (calms)
- Chamomile Tea
- Anise Tea (gas relief)

MELATONIN RICH FOODS:

- Pure cherry juice
- Scottish/Irish oatmeal* [1/2 cup for adults and adolescents; 1/4 cup for children]

OTHER CALMING FOODS:

- Bananas ($\downarrow$ BP with $\uparrow$ potassium)
- Honey (glucose $\downarrow$ OREXIN that $\uparrow$ alertness)
- Non-alcoholic beer ($\uparrow$ GABA, a brain tranquilizer)
- $\uparrow$ Magnesium to $\downarrow$ sweating (check with MD for levels needed)
- Cinnamon or nutmeg (added to foods $\uparrow$ calming, muscle-relaxing alpha brain waves)
- Wheat germ ($\uparrow$ B_6 Vit.)

NOTES:_____

_____

_____

_____

_____

BEDTIME ROUTINE

Name: _____ Week of: __/__/_____

TIME	ACTIVITY	NOTES
	• Light snack 1 hour before bath time	
	• Take a warm water bath/shower	
	• Put on relaxing pajamas	
	• Brush teeth with warm/tepid water	
	• Go to bathroom/potty	
	• Make room quiet & comfortable, cooler better than warmer…lights dim or off	
	• Read/look at book or listen to music/ book in "womb" area with small light	
	• Unwind ½ to 1 hour before actual bedtime using 1 or more of the following strategies: 1._____ 2._____ 3._____ 4._____	
	• Say "Good night" & leave at bedtime.	

DAY	COMMENTS	CHANGES
Monday		
Tuesday		
Wednesday		
Thursday		
Friday		
Saturday		
Sunday		

LEGEND: √ Done as listed. Overall Reaction: + = Positive, 0 = No Impact, - = Negative

AUTISM SLEEPS

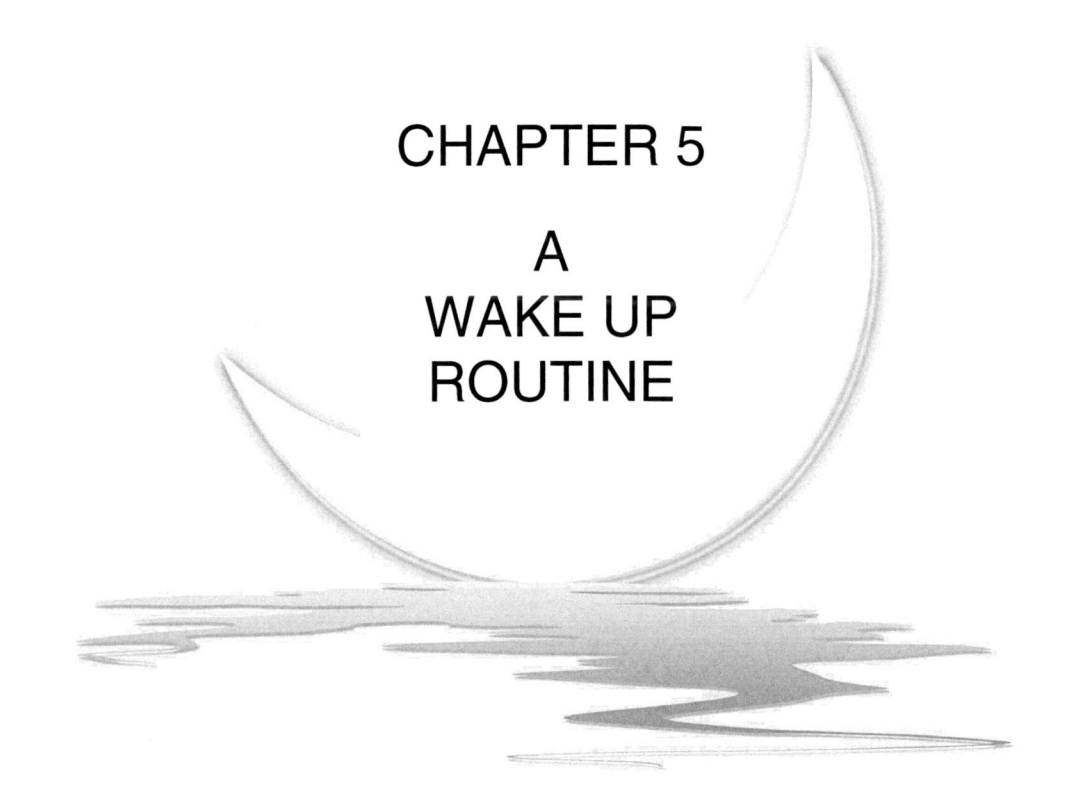

CHAPTER 5

A
WAKE UP
ROUTINE

AUTISM SLEEPS

SAMPLE WAKE UP SCHEDULE

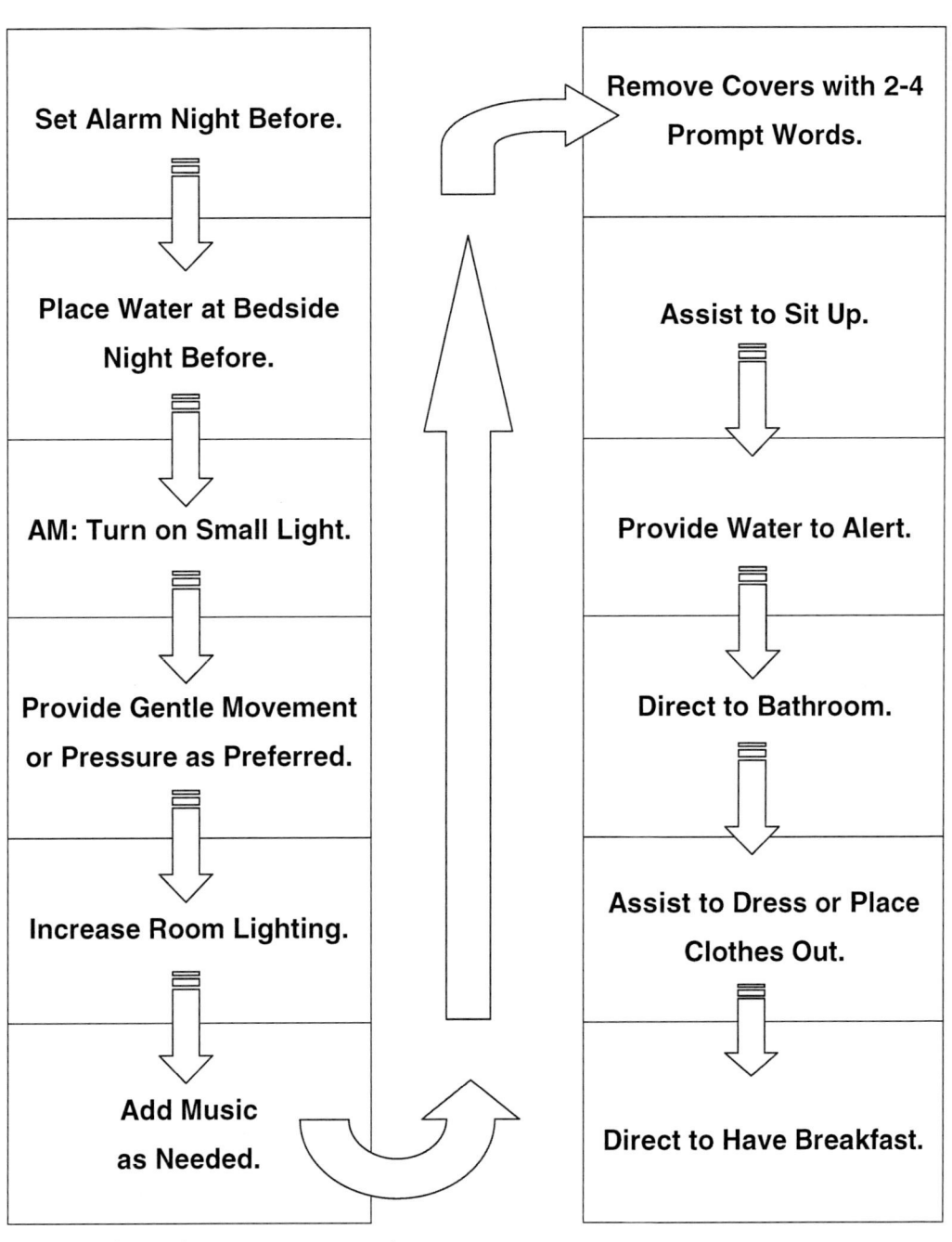

Set Alarm Night Before.

Place Water at Bedside Night Before.

AM: Turn on Small Light.

Provide Gentle Movement or Pressure as Preferred.

Increase Room Lighting.

Add Music as Needed.

Remove Covers with 2-4 Prompt Words.

Assist to Sit Up.

Provide Water to Alert.

Direct to Bathroom.

Assist to Dress or Place Clothes Out.

Direct to Have Breakfast.

WAKE UP ROUTINE & STRATEGIES

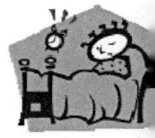

If the person is sensitive or irritable usually upon awakening, try one or more of the following sensory strategies:

- ☐ Place a flowering plant on the bed stand to increase visual alertness & to have oxygen source for added brain health.

- ☐ Gently rock in slow, small movements while in side-lying position in bed with one hand on the shoulder & one on the hip, gradually increasing in movement.

- ☐ Provide gentle pressure, gradually becoming lighter, on the forehead &/or cheeks—areas of high sensitivity.

- ☐ Play graduated music, increasing volume slowly until at the level that awakens.

- ☐ Use graduated full spectrum lighting to brighten room slowly until full brightness is achieved— some alarms are programmable to do this automatically.

- ☐ Drink a glass of filtered, mineralized and ionized water at room temperature to initially hydrate to awaken/orient the brain to a state of balance or homeostasis.

- ☐ Eat a food with protein within 30 minutes of awakening.

WAKE UP ROUTINE & STRATEGIES

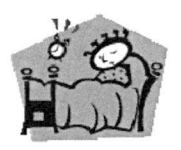

If the person is very *difficult to awaken* or a *heavy sleeper*, try one or more of the following sensory strategies:

- ☐ Set a loud, large alarm that repeats until pressed, placed across the room to require leaving the bed to be turned off.

- ☐ Remove socks or, if feet are bare, place a cool to cold cloth on one or both to increase body's alerting system.

- ☐ Have a graduated, full spectrum lamp that can be programmed to full brightness when alarm is activated or turn on a full spectrum lamp to full brightness before awakening verbally.

- ☐ Provide a drink of cool to cold water to increase brain hydration while increasing alertness.

- ☐ Remove or pull back covers if wrapped up to arouse with cooler overall body temperature.

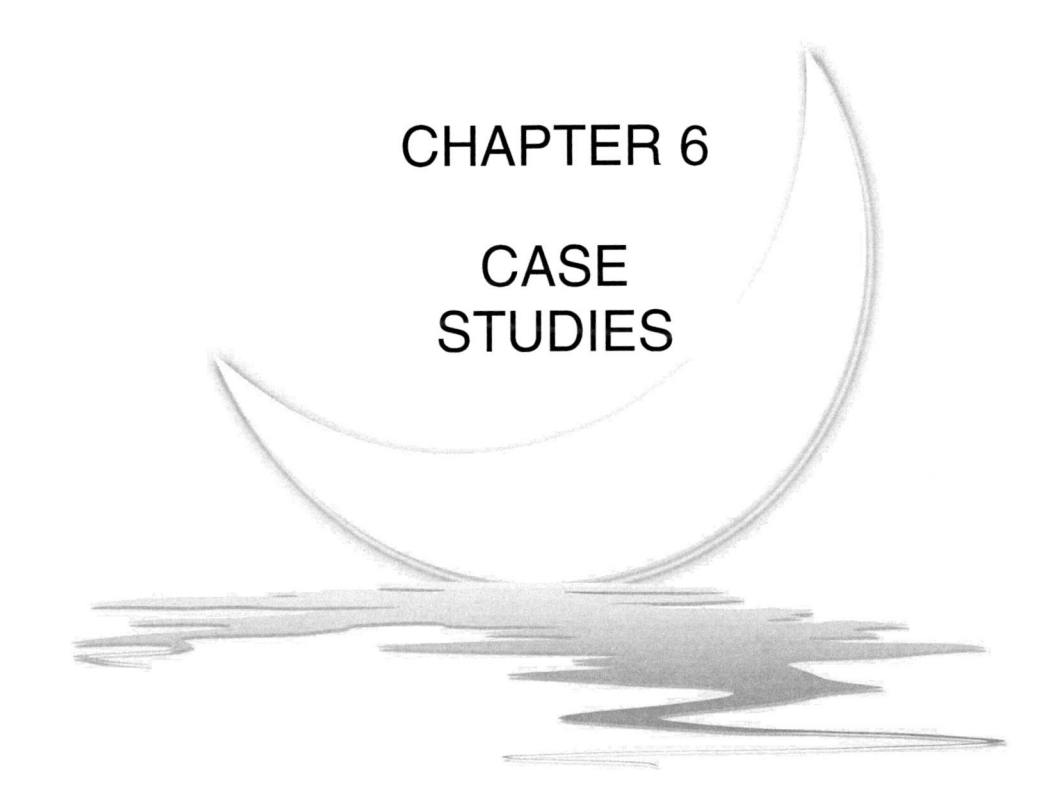

CHAPTER 6

CASE
STUDIES

CASE STUDIES

#1 CHILD: Aiden

Aiden is a 4-year-old boy that was reported to have sensory processing difficulties during an evaluation at the local public school system. His mother, Brenda, reported typical problem behaviors that included hitting, biting, screaming, slapping, running away, not listening to directives given and difficulty sharing in his preschool classes. These are frequent behaviors that also occur with children with an Autism Spectrum Disorder. At the point that he was referred to this therapist, Aiden had been expelled from two private preschools. His parents were awaiting recommendations from the public school system regarding assistance and options that could be provided through the Special Education services at a more appropriate placement.

Being the first child and grandchild in the family, his parents, Brenda and Brian, had not had formalized training on discipline strategies that are typically needed with children exhibiting sensory-based problem behaviors. Brenda was referred to this therapist for assistance with Aiden's sensory processing difficulties to improve his behaviors.

The first evaluation session involved an evaluation to determine the root of the behaviors, as well as Aiden's reaction to his overall home environment. This is the first area in a child's life where behaviors like these typically develop. Through review of the school arena report where multiple disciplines assessed him simultaneously, the *Pediatric Evaluation Scale (PES)* indicated that he presented with above average scores in all developmental areas, except for Personal-Social skills that were significantly lower and below average. Though Aiden is a very bright,

CASE STUDIES (Continued)—

#1 CHILD: Aiden

intelligent little boy, he lacked self-regulation or the ability to manage his emotions to properly interact with his peers or adults around him.

Within 10 minutes of this therapist's arrival to the home, Aiden began screaming, throwing himself on the floor and slapping his mother instead of following his mother's instruction to sit quietly so she could speak with this therapist. After a quick history of his sensory concerns, this therapist approached Aiden to attempt to intervene. He immediately began slapping this therapist and screaming. This therapist picked up his feet and asked him to "walk on your hands" to go to his seat. He refused to "walk", fisting his hands and flexing his body to avoid moving forward. With the help of his mother, he was placed in a vertical position with his head hanging mid-air to calm him using inversion that typically lowers blood pressure. This therapist kept her legs apart since he continuously grabbed them and tried to bite them. His mother assisted to keep Aiden free from this therapist, and to place him upstairs on the carpet for his safety. (He was lying on hardwood floors downstairs previously, and could have been hurt from his flailing movements.)

Upstairs, Aiden's mother held his arms to keep him from hitting and pinching while this therapist crossed his legs and kept them flexed to keep him from kicking. He had to be stabilized at his pelvis to keep from sliding out from this position. The prompt words, "When you are quiet, you can go to your room," were stated each time Aiden lashed out verbally screaming, "I AM THE BOSS!" The mother was asked to get the therapist's "special"

CASE STUDIES (Continued)—

#1 CHILD: Aiden

SPORT water bottle and a cup to give Aiden some "Magic water". Brenda provided these items, and poured filtered, mineralized and ionized water from the SPORT bottle into the cup. At first Aiden would not accept it, but after Brenda was asked to go downstairs to take a break and get some water herself, he agreed to drink. (At this point Brenda was nearly in tears watching her son for approximately 40 minutes in a state of rage and out of control, almost appearing to be "possessed" per her comments.) Within 5 seconds of drinking the water, Aiden asked this therapist, "Could you please count to 10 again so I can stop crying and calm down?" Very willing to do so, the slow, methodical counting began from 1 to 10 during which time Aiden held his crying with great difficulty and eventually quieted at reaching "10". He was told, "Now that you are quiet and calm, you can go to your room." Aiden then stood up, and walked to his room quietly and very calmly. On reaching his room, he asked this therapist if he could read a book to her, and immediately sat on the floor to attempt to sound out words based on pictures on each page. He readily accepted assistance to sound out the words, and stayed in his room, even after the therapist left to go downstairs to continue the evaluation and combination training session with his mother.

On reaching the downstairs dining area, Brenda asked, "Where is Aiden? It's as if he is another child!" She was amazed at how quiet he was. In analysis of the sensory input that was provided, Aiden responded to deep pressure (proprioceptive-joint input), inversion by being held upside down or vertically (vestibular input-movement input), consistent verbal prompts

CASE STUDIES (Continued)—

#1 CHILD: Aiden

(auditory-heard input) and oral input by drinking water that hydrates the brain and serves as a universal sensory strategy to either increase alertness or calm agitation, as needed.

Once Aiden was calm and playing alone in his room, the session continued with completion of a behavioral rating scale and an analysis of Aiden's day which included his sleep behavior history. Additionally, his room environment was assessed. The colors on the walls were bright red on the lower half with white walls on the upper half that included a wide, black border along the perimeter of the walls closest to the ceiling. There was a wall mural of Thomas the Train in bright red, blues, white and black with very stark, bright, contrasting colors which are not conducive for calming and relaxation. Additionally, a full body-sized figure of Iron Man was standing in the room just below the foot of the bed at the wall, staring at the bed area which could elicit images of monsters or strangers in the room in the dark. When asked if Aiden had commented about being fearful in his room, Brenda reported that he had already asked to have Thomas taken off his wall several times. There was a train alphabet with separate cards of the letters of the alphabet on the far wall from the bed, adding to the high contrast, bright colors and distracters in the room. On one angled side of the ceiling, there were stenciled sports balls filling the entire area in a busy pattern. There was a small bookcase and a bench at the foot of the bed in front of the window, and a small lamp on the dresser next to the bed in addition to a night light. In the other room there was a glider that was used

CASE STUDIES (Continued)—

#1 CHILD: Aiden

when Aiden was a baby that was not currently in use. Brenda also relayed that his room was his "Time out" area for Aiden to retreat when he was misbehaving.

Based on the above assessment of his room environment, the following recommendations were made. His parents were suggested to:

1. Remove Thomas the Train and the Iron Man figures;
2. Replace the red lower walls with a more neutral or calming color (tan, for example);
3. Change the upper white wall color to a soothing blue in a more pale tone, such as periwinkle, sky blue, etc.;
4. Remove the bench and replace it with the glider in the corner for Aiden to self-calm, as needed, and to incorporate it into his Preparatory sensory strategies for his bedtime routine;
5. Rearrange the bed to be able to access it from both sides and make the room more accessible;
6. Remove the sports stencils on the ceiling and paint the ceiling with a more neutral color;
7. Transfer the alphabet train for placement in a linear pattern (as the train cars would be aligned), but along the wide, black border that followed at the top of the walls along the ceiling for three sides in front of the bed;
8. Place room-darkening shades or curtains;
9. Keep a glass of "Magic water" at the bedside for use on awakening;

CASE STUDIES (Continued)—

#1-CHILD: Aiden

10. Add background noise through the use of a portable air filter to also clean the room air;
11. Add a graduated light with full spectrum lighting to simulate sunrise for assistance with awakening, and sunset with calming on low as a Preparatory Strategy, and
12. Place a magnetic topper, pillow and comforter on the standard full-sized mattress as a Functional Sensory Strategy to help Aiden's entire body to calm into a deeper level of sleep.

This therapist provided a magnetic mattress topper, pillow and comforter, and placed it on the left side of the bed where Aiden usually sleeps. Aiden immediately got between the covers, which Brenda stated he usually never uses, and lied on his back stating, "This is comfortable!" A large container of "Magic" water was also provided for use throughout the day, especially two hours prior to bedtime to hydrate Aiden's body and brain with pure, mineralized and ionized water to help him hydrate and further calm. Additionally, other recommendations were made, and a copy of the forms of this book were provided to guide Aiden's parents as to the sensory strategies that could/should be used, as well as the routines for getting to bed/sleep and for awakening.

To address the other sensory-based problem areas, a ball chair (made from inverting a thick-walled, large ball and inflating it inside a heavy-duty crate) was provided for Aiden to increase sitting in front of the television to provide the input he appeared to seek from the need for movement.

CASE STUDIES (Continued)—

#1-CHILD: Aiden

Though a wedge-shaped cushion was tried on the dining room chair to increase Aiden's sitting time at the table, the chair itself did not provide the postural or positioning support Aiden needed to be stabilized in sitting. Brenda stated that she would replace the booster seat that could be connected to the chair to give Aiden the continued support he still appeared to need, particularly to help with table time sitting with the family.

By the time this therapist and Brenda returned downstairs and Aiden rejoined them, he was hugging and kissing this therapist, seeking the attention of both now. He was told, "When you say, 'Excuse me', and ask permission to speak, then we will answer you." Aiden did not automatically do this until a hand was held up on his approach with prompting to use this phrase without eye contact to reinforce his interruptions. After several trials, he learned the prompts and repeatedly asked for permission as directed. He also stayed in the living room playing with his toys while the training session was completed with his mother.

Brenda was given a prompt sheet that delineated the Behavior Continuum Theory, as outlined in a publication authored by this therapist called, *The Scale of Sensory Strategies (SOSS) Toolkit®*. The sensory strategies utilized were recorded on the *S.O.S.S.* Long Form A data collection sheet to keep track of the impact of each for future use or avoidance. She was also trained on the *H-A-L-T Principle* that this therapist uses to initially assess the root of behaviors. Could they be because Aiden was Hungry, Angry, Lonely or Tired? Based on the response(s) to this, the appropriate sensory-based versus cognitively-based strategies could be implemented.

CASE STUDIES (Continued)—

#1-CHILD: Aiden

Two days after visiting Aiden for the first time, Brenda was contacted to determine how he was doing. Aiden usually slept seven to eight hours a day with awakening several times during the night, whining or complaining in the morning on arising. The first night on the sleep system with use of the water only, Aiden slept 11 hours and did not awaken during the night. Four days later the pattern continued with Aiden awakening in a positive and happy mood in the mornings per his mother. As a result, the other behavior strategies recommended have been more easily implemented with improved mood and attitude.

#2-ADOLESCENT: Kevin

Kevin is an 18 year old high school Senior who attends the local public school. He receives Special Education services via placement in a Mild Intellectual Disabilities classroom for sensory-motor support and specialized academic instruction through an Individualized Education Plan or IEP. He was initially referred to this therapist at the early age of 6 years for having difficulties with handwriting and overall fine motor control. He also exhibited difficulties in several of the sensory processing areas, particularly for a sensory-based motor disorder or dyspraxia with significant difficulty for gross and fine motor sequencing.

For many years this therapist worked with Kevin and his parents, Angela and Mike, privately. Then he was added to this therapist's public school

CASE STUDIES (Continued)—

#2-ADOLESCENT: Kevin

caseload, so his private therapy services were discontinued until the end of 5th grade when he was then transferred to another therapist in middle school. At that point this therapist continued working with Kevin and his parents only on an ongoing and as-needed basis, primarily as a consultant for any additional higher level home activities of daily living, as well as for recommendations on possible needs for his school-based services. This therapist also was given permission by Angela and Mike to collaborate with the school-based Occupational Therapist in order to coordinate sensory and motor strategies that could be used in both settings.

Many sensory areas were addressed and a wide variety of strategies or interventions were implemented in the home and school settings respectively. These include dietary considerations since Kevin was allergic to eggs, gluten and dairy products; therefore, his parents strictly watched what he ate. Ultimately, Kevin was also taught how to determine which foods he could eat, and restricted himself, as well.

Another area of particular need was for Kevin's continued toe walking. Given that this was not an area addressed in the school system, this therapist recommended the use of shoe weights to give Kevin the Proprioceptive or joint pressure input he seemed to be seeking when he bounced on the balls of his feet while walking. As the need for shoe weights was explained to his parents, Mike agreed that this might help. However, Mike's understanding, as an engineer, was that the weights would be added to the heels to pull his feet down flat. When the shoe

CASE STUDIES (Continued)—

#2-ADOLESCENT: Kevin

weights arrived, this therapist attached them on top of the front end of the shoes over the ball of each foot, secured by the intermingled lacing. Mike gazed at the shoes and this therapist, and displayed a look of great puzzlement. Then, when Kevin took his first steps and his gait pattern was as typical as that of his father's, Mike really looked bewildered. On being unable to understand how this type of input could possibly work, he commented in amazement to this therapist, "I don't see how that can work! That just doesn't seem logical!" To that, this therapist then replied, "You're right, Mike. It's NOT logical, it's *NEURO*logical!" This therapist then explained that some reactions cannot be easily explained because the root of the original problems are not always obvious or "logical". With that explanation, Mike and Angela were religious with their follow-through for using the shoe weights, and helped Kevin obtain a typical gait pattern after several months. They were always consistent and faithful about following this therapist's suggested interventions, even when the justification for the therapy strategies did not seem "logical"!

In the case of a sleep problem, the interventions needed might also be NEUROlogical (brain-based). However, they could also be ENDOCRINOlogical (hormone-based), PSYCHOlogical (mentally-based), BIOlogical (dealing with internal systems) or PHYSIOlogical (musculo-skeletal based)….depending on the root of the sleep difficulties, especially in the case of a person with atypical sensory processing.

As the years progressed, sleep began to become a problem as Kevin approached puberty. He began waking in the early or middle part of the

CASE STUDIES (Continued)—

#2-ADOLESCENT: Kevin

morning, going downstairs on the main level of the home, and staying awake the rest of the morning until it was time to go to school. Needless to say, his school performance was not progressing as preferred by his parents and his teachers. His parents had already tried several sensory strategies since their repertoire of sensory interventions from many years of therapy had made them "honorary O.T.'s" per this therapist's opinion. They had placed a Salt Rock in Kevin's room to help with calming, as well as his breathing. They had also added a fan for background or "white" noise to help Kevin relax in getting himself ready for sleep. The walls were painted in a soothing blue tone and he had a night light and bedside lamp for a sense of security as needed. Additionally, his parents bought him a set of Bose headphones and sound system. He very much enjoyed listening to talk radio that was very soothing to Kevin to mentally relax. There was also no television or computer in his room to visually distract him and visually stimulate him at bedtime.

When this therapist was contacted to consult regarding helping Kevin stay asleep to enable more restful, healthy sleep, a suggestion was made to have Kevin begin drinking filtered, mineralized and ionized water throughout the day until about 2 hours before bedtime. His parents were then given a magnetic sleep system on loan with magnets embedded in the mattress topper, the pillow and the comforter. Kevin had been sleeping no more than 6-7 hours at that time when he needed a minimum of 9 hours each night. He generally removed his covers due to heavy sweating and

CASE STUDIES (Continued)—

#2-ADOLESCENT: Kevin

was having increased difficulty with sustained focus in school, especially for his 1-Minute Math trials. Much to his parents' surprise after the first night on the magnetic sleep system, Kevin slept a little over 11 hours. His parents even went into his room to be sure he was breathing and not having any problems when he was not awake on that Saturday morning, as he typically would be watching television or playing his video games. Kevin also reported that he slept really well, and did not sweat throughout the night. His acne also improved after several days and weeks of reduced or no sweating to irritate his facial skin surface.

Since the sleep system provided the benefits of magnetic energy to help Kevin's body relax itself during the night, he also needed a daytime system to help him with his mental and physical demands. He used a magnetic necklace on a daily basis. The first day a magnetic neck band was placed on Kevin, he remarked, "I can think better now!" Whether that was fact or not, in his perception it was true. The real proof of this was when the magnetic insoles were added into his school athletic shoes that he wore daily. His mother did not send a note or tell the teacher that morning that she had inserted insoles into his shoes to see if there would be a true change in his abilities. That afternoon after Kevin returned from school and his parents got home, Angela read a note from his teacher that said, "Kevin was calmer and focused today, and got a 100 on his Math quiz!" [Generally, Kevin's best scores were between 60 and 70 percentiles at best.]

CASE STUDIES (Continued)—

#2-ADOLESCENT: Kevin

Kevin also wore a magnetic headband after school prior to shooting basketball hoops at home. He stated emphatically that this helped him to improve his "game", as well.

To date, after approximately one and one-half years of using his sensory sleep strategies and the magnetic sleep system, Kevin's sleep pattern continues to be a healthy one. As reported by his mother, he sleeps for longer uninterrupted periods of time, awakening early less often at an average of only once monthly. During school days he goes to bed at 9:00 and is awakened at 5:30 to get ready for the bus ride. On weekends and holidays, or when he is not required to awaken at a specific time, he still sleeps approximately 11 hours or more. He is still not sweating at night, does not snore and awakens in a good mood, appearing rested to tackle his day.

Kevin also still, "Loves his insoles," per Angela. She explained that he likes the way the insoles make him feel, and will automatically transfer them from his athletic to other shoes as needed without prompting. He also continues to wear his neck band daily and drink his "special" water from his SPORT bottle throughout his day to, "..give him energy!" Additionally, his basketball game has greatly improved, shooting "ringers" quite regularly into the hoops while wearing his magnetic headband. Overall, Kevin continues to experience a pattern of healthy sleep as he benefits from the impact of his sensory sleep strategies as provided by his parents.

CASE STUDIES (Continued)—

#3-ADULT: Blake

Blake was a little boy diagnosed with a severe Autism Spectrum Disorder (ASD) at the young age of two and a half years. He was served by this therapist in the home initially to intervene and manage very challenging sensory-based problem behaviors to prepare him to transition to school. He entered the local public elementary school to begin attending a modified day in a Special Education class for children with severe ASD. His time was gradually increased until he tolerated attending a full day for the remainder of his elementary school years. However, when he reached puberty and entered middle school, he required more intensive instruction and interventions for severe sensory and cognitively-based problem behaviors. At that point he required placement at a local center that specialized in the management of persons with ASD. He continued at this center for the duration of time through high school until his "graduation" from the local public school system when he turned 22 years of age.

Blake had significant digestive issues. Though he was never a picky eater, as is typical with many persons with Autism, his parents, Claire and Mark, controlled his intake in an attempt to help him with his stomach problems. He was ultimately placed on a gluten and casein free diet that helped significantly. Prior to this diet change, his head banging would be exacerbated whenever he ate foods made from wheat. It was not until Claire discovered a vegetable-based enzyme that his digestive problems became manageable and under control.

At the age of 13 years, after the worst of puberty had passed per his mother, Blake began having significantly more difficulty sleeping. For an

CASE STUDIES (Continued)—

#3-ADULT: Blake

entire year he was unable to sleep more than six hours maximum per night for only one to two nights in a full week. In addition to his sleep difficulties, the lack of sleep amplified his problem behaviors in the home and school environments. Claire and Mark tried many strategies to help his quality and quantity of sleep. Blake was kept on a regular schedule due to his need for routine in his day where exercise and a high intake of water were integral. Though no specific foods were used to prepare for bedtime, he was not allowed any liquids after dinner time. He was also not given any rewards or positive reinforcement if he awoke during the night, but simply returned to his bed. Blake's parents, Claire and Mark, have an in-depth knowledge of Autism, and Blake's bedroom environment was made to be very conducive to relaxation and self-calming. The room was constructed without windows to make it totally dark at night. The walls were painted with a deep tan color without any hangings for optimum relaxation. There were no toys in the room or other distracters. An air purifier was used to not only provide clean air to facilitate breathing, but to serve as a "white" or background noise for further calming. Additionally, a rocker recliner was the only piece of furniture in the room other than the full-sized bed. So, if Blake ever was to awaken at night to use the bathroom, his attendant would guide him to the recliner to prepare for bed again or directly back to the bed to try to return to sleep. Even with all these strategies in place, nothing seemed to be helping during this very challenging period.

It was not until Blake's parents met a woman from Macon, Georgia, who suggested a magnetic sleep system that his sleep issues became

CASE STUDIES (Continued)—

#3-ADULT: Blake

manageable. She suggested a trial period of one week using a sleep system embedded with magnets that included a mattress topper, a comforter and a natural latex pillow to help Blake get into a deeper state of sleep. His parents agreed, and the woman drove to the home in Duluth, Georgia, to provide the trial sleep system. By the end of the one-week trial period, Blake had slept an average of eight hours every night. The impact of this sensory strategy was so dramatic, that the entire family began sleeping on these magnetic systems, and continue to this day. Even Mark, who snored and had difficulty falling asleep, snored less and was able to sleep throughout the night!

Blake continued to use the magnetic sleep system without any sleep interruption other than waking once a night every two to three weeks on average to the age of 23. The only time during this period that he exhibited problem sleep behaviors was when he began a trial of Hyperbaric Oxygen treatment. Blake was placed for one hour per day into an oxygen chamber in an attempt to improve his overall cognitive abilities that were significantly impacted by his Autism. Though his level of alertness and attention significantly improved per Claire, Blake's agitation increased drastically, and he had difficulty breathing with poor sleep quality once again. Overall, it was reportedly a very bad experience though his parents' understanding was that this had helped other persons with Autism. Their belief is that this may have occurred due to the interaction of the high intake levels of

CASE STUDIES (Continued)—

#3-ADULT: Blake

oxygen that perhaps interacted negatively with the side effects of the many medications Blake was taking.

Blake's sleep quality and length of sleep became so compromised that he required the need for sleep medications for a short time until he could be regulated back to his prior level of function. At that point his parents were able to return to use of the routine sensory sleep strategies that were in place prior to this interruption. Blake then returned and benefited from a pattern of continuous, quality sleep thereafter.

AUTISM SLEEPS

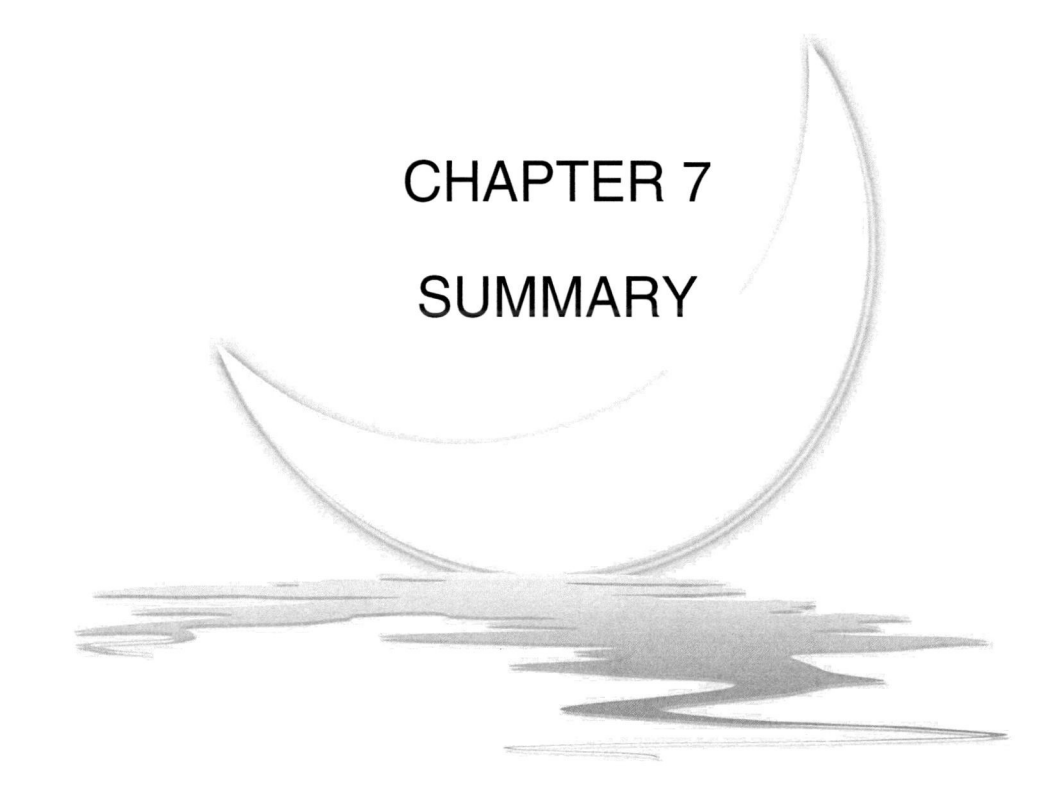

CHAPTER 7

SUMMARY

	Mon	Tues	Wed	Th	Fri	Sat	Sun
(time)_____ Unwind Before Bed							
Take a bath							
Put pajamas on							
Have an evening snack							
(time)_____ Get Ready For Bed							
Brush Teeth							
Read							
(time)_____ Go To Bed							

SUMMARY

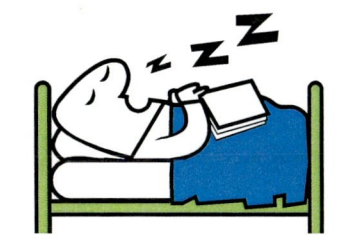

❖ Make bedtime a **POSITIVE ACTIVITY** that the individual will look forward to experiencing. Keep the bedroom as a positive place—not a "time out" or area for punishment.

❖ Be **CONSISTENT** with bedtimes in order to establish a true **ROUTINE**—With children, do not negotiate where to sleep; follow the path of most resistance, if this is an issue, by not giving in to crying or whining to change beds during the night.

❖ Utilize a variety of **PREPARATORY SENSORY STRATEGIES** to help get the person ready to sleep; **FUNCTIONAL SENSORY STRATEGIES** to get and keep the sleeper in a state of relaxation; and **TRANSITIONAL SENSORY STRATEGIES** to enable the sleeper to wake up without startling or jolting the nervous system abruptly.

SUMMARY [Continued]—

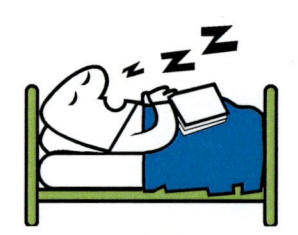

Practice the *4 B's (B4) Before Bedtime*:

1. ***B*ATH....Draw a warm, aromatic *BATH* to cleanse/relax & to play with tub toys to wind down for children;**

2. ***B*OOK....Read or look at a *BOOK* to gear down mentally;**

3. ***B*ATHROOM....GO to avoid waking;**

4. ***B*EAR HUG....Give a *BEAR or BODY HUG* as tolerated to say, "Good night & sweet dreams!"**

Good night...

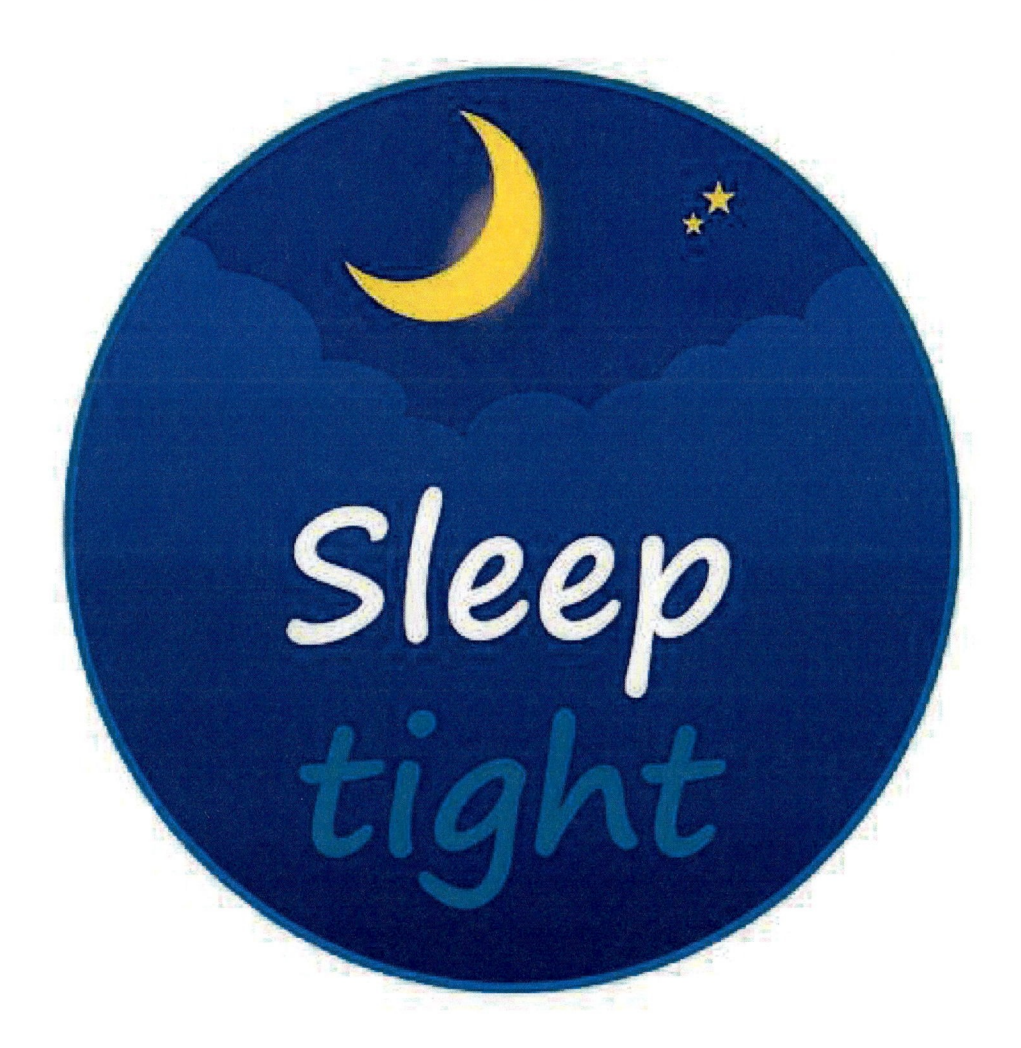

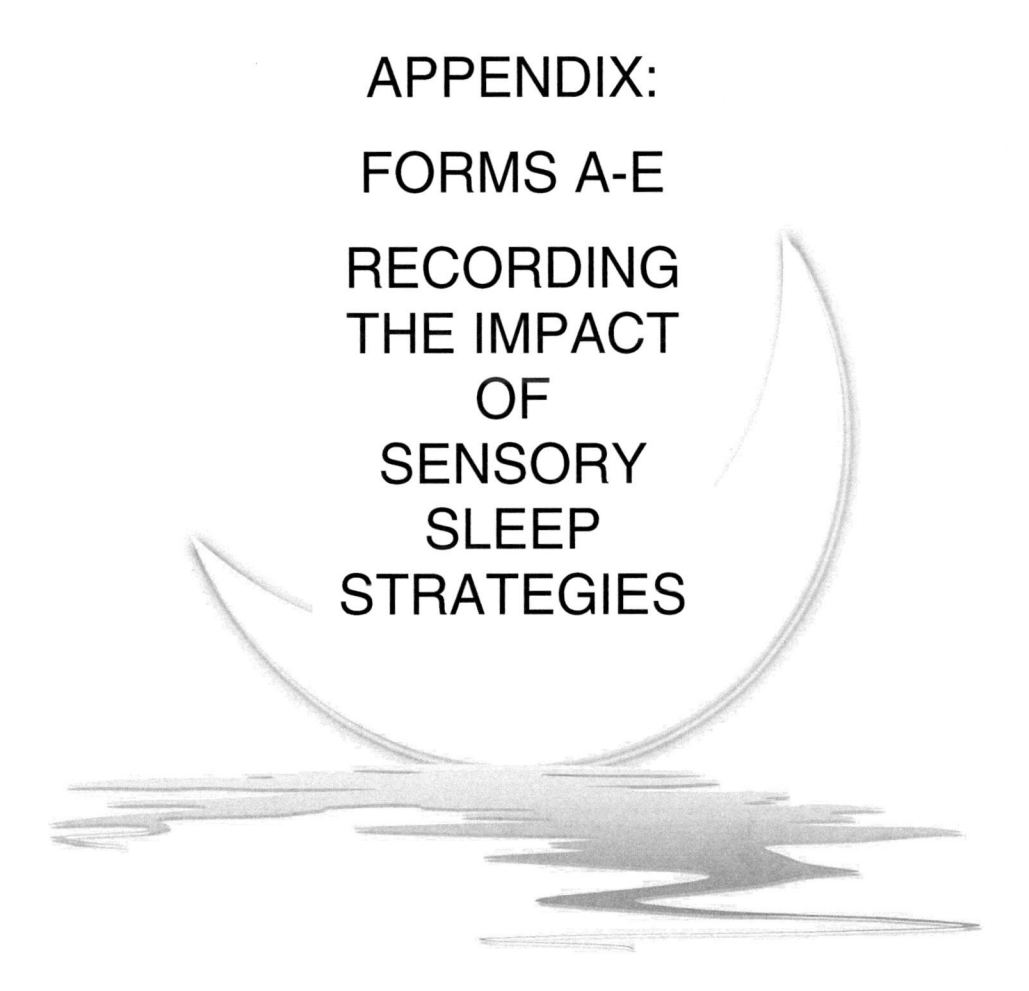

APPENDIX:

FORMS A-E

RECORDING
THE IMPACT
OF
SENSORY
SLEEP
STRATEGIES

FORM A-1:   BEDTIME ROUTINE

Name: _____ Week of: __/__/_____

TIME	ACTIVITY	NOTES
	• Light snack 1 hour before bath time	
	• Take a warm water bath/ shower	
	• Put on relaxing pajamas	
	• Brush teeth with warm/tepid water	
	• Go to bathroom/potty	
	• Make room quiet & comfortable, cooler better than warmer… lights dim or off	
	• Read/look at book or listen to music/ book in "womb" area with small light	
	• Unwind ½ to 1 hour before actual bed-time using 1 or more of the following strategies: 1._____ 2._____ 3._____ 4._____	
	• Say "Good night" & leave at bedtime.	

DAY	COMMENTS	CHANGES
Monday		
Tuesday		
Wednesday		
Thursday		
Friday		
Saturday		
Sunday		

LEGEND: √ Done as listed.   Overall Reaction : + = Positive, 0 = No Impact, - = Negative

AUTISM SLEEPS

FORM B-1:   SENSORY SLEEP STRATEGIES CHECKLIST

Period: _____ to _____

SENSORY AREA: [Touch / Tactile Sense]

Skin

- ☐ Warm __ bath or __ shower 1 hour before bedtime
- ☐ Foot rub or massage
- ☐ Face --gentle massage
- ☐ Back rub or vibrating massager
- ☐ Palm pressure at temples
- ☐ Forehead/ temple rubs
- ☐ Lotion on __ arms __ legs
- ☐ Brushing or stroking hair
- ☐ Cool room temperature
- ☐ __ Loose or __ snug pajamas
- ☐ Holding pet or stuffed animal

SENSORY AREA: [Respiration / Olfactory Sense]

Lungs

- ☐ Air purification system that filters/ cleans & ionizes
- ☐ Nasal / personal inhaler
- ☐ Other: _____
- ☐ Open nasal passages if congested (Saline spray/cool mist vaporizer)
- ☐ Walk or light exercise 1 hour+ before bedtime for 5 minutes or less

Aromatherapy with *essential oils* to open airways & relax/ calm:
- ☐ Eucalyptus ☐ Peppermint ☐ Tea Tree ☐ Cinnamon ☐ Lavender

SENSORY AREA: [Sight / Visual Sense]

Eyes

- ☐ Picture schedule for routine
- ☐ Night light [warm tones]
- ☐ Salt Rock or Lava Lamp
- ☐ Read or look at a book
- ☐ Dimmed or rope lighting
- ☐ Corner or bed tent "womb" area
- ☐ ↓ Distracters (stimulating items)
- ☐ Slow or static ceiling projection
- ☐ Other: _____

SENSORY AREA: [Hearing / Auditory Sense]

Ears

- ☐ White noise machine or fan
- ☐ Listen to a book or a CD
- ☐ Ear plugs or headphones
- ☐ Nature sounds— waterfall, ocean waves, wind, crickets, etc. (recorded or electronic)
- ☐ Classical music [< 60 beats per min.]*
- ☐ Soothing music or Metronome *
- ☐ Other: _____

SENSORY AREA: [Joints & Movement / Vestibular & Proprioceptive Sense]

Position

- ☐ "Womb" area- beanbag lying 30 min. before bed
- ☐ Glider rocking 30 min. prior
- ☐ Multiple sleeping bags
- ☐ Percussion on back
- ☐ Gentle rocking in bed
- ☐ Stuffed animals to hug
- ☐ Multiple bed pillows
- ☐ Calming/ Magnetic Sleep System
- ☐ Body pillow to "spoon"/hug
- ☐ Weighted blanket/ "snake"/ toys
- ☐ Other: _____

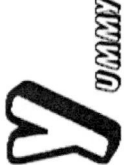

SENSORY AREA: [Eating or Drinking / Oral or Gustatory Sense] Period: _____ to _____

MELATONIN RICH Foods:

☐ Pure cherry juice

☐ Scottish/ Irish oatmeal*
[1/2 cup for adults
adolescents; 1/4 cup for
children]

TRYPTOPHAN RICH Foods:

☐ Cottage & other cheeses

☐ Chew Chia seeds (2 Tbsp.)

☐ Peanuts/Peanut butter

☐ Sesame seeds/butter

☐ Milk—Warm or tepid

☐ Pineapples, plums

☐ Turkey patty, etc.

☐ Sunflower seeds

☐ Popcorn-Light

☐ Oatmeal *

☐ Pudding

☐ Yogurt

☐ Eggs

DETOXIFICATION AID:

☐ WATER—3 hours before
bed & on awakening
[Filtered, mineralized &
Ionized—most hydrating]

☐

DIGESTIVE AIDS:

☐ Cumin Seeds (↓gas,
bloating & discomfort)

☐ Valerian Tea (sedative)

☐ Tilia (Tilo) Tea (calming)

☐ Anise Tea (gas relief)

☐ Chamomile Tea

☐

☐

☐

☐

☐

OTHER CALMING FOODS:

☐ Bananas (↓ BP with ↑ potassium)

☐ Honey (glucose ↓ OREXIN that ↑
alertness)

☐ Non-alcoholic beer (↑ GABA, a brain
tranquilizer)

☐ ↑ Magnesium to ↓ sweating (check
with physician for levels needed)

☐ Cinnamon, nutmeg or vanilla (added to
foods ↑ calming, muscle-relaxing
alpha brain waves)

☐ Wheat germ (↑ Vitamin B_6)

☐

☐

☐

☐

☐

☐

☐

NOTES:

_____

_____

_____

FORM D-1: SLEEP RECORD

Page ___

Name: _____ Month: _____ Year: _____ Baseline: _____ Hours

No.	Day	Sleep Strategy*	Time Used	A M	P M	Time Asleep	A M	P M	Time Awake	A M	P M	Times Awakened	Hours Slept	IMPACT (Hours) ⇩	√ NO CHANGE	⇧

| | = TOTAL NUMBER OF DAYS | | | TOTAL IMPACT IN HOURS: | -- | + |

SUM OF IMPACT = [ ]   / SUM OF DAYS = AVERAGE CHANGE: [ ]

* NOTE: Try one sensory or schedule change strategy at a time to isolate impact or effect on any possible behavioral changes.

FORM E-1: SLEEP RECORD GRAPH

Name: _____   Sleep Period: ___/___/_____ to ___/___/_____

HOURS	Day 1	Day 2	Day 3	Day 4	Day 5	Day 6	Day 7	Day 8	Day 9	Day 10	Day 11	Day 12	Day 13	Day 14
10														
9														
8														
7														
6														
5														
4														
3														
2														
1														
0														
-1														
-2														
-3														
-4														
-5														
-6														
-7														
-8														
-9														
-10														

FORM A-2: BEDTIME ROUTINE

Name: _____ Week of: __/__/_____

TIME	ACTIVITY	NOTES
	• Light snack 1 hour before bath time	
	• Take a warm water bath/shower	
	• Put on relaxing pajamas	
	• Brush teeth with warm/tepid water	
	• Go to bathroom/ potty	
	• Make room quiet & comfortable, cooler better than warmer… lights dim or off	
	• Read/look at book or listen to music/ book in "womb" area with small light	
	• Unwind ½ to 1 hour before actual bedtime using 1 or more of the following strategies: 1._____ 2._____ 3._____ 4._____	
	• Say "Good night" & leave at bedtime.	

DAY	COMMENTS	CHANGES
Monday		
Tuesday		
Wednesday		
Thursday		
Friday		
Saturday		
Sunday		

LEGEND: √ Done as listed. Overall Reaction : + = Positive, 0 = No Impact, - = Negative

SENSORY SLEEP STRATEGIES CHECKLIST

Period: _____ to _____

SENSORY AREA: [Touch / Tactile Sense]

SKIN

- ☐ Warm __ bath or __ shower 1 hour before bedtime
- ☐ Foot rub or massage
- ☐ Face --gentle massage
- ☐ Back rub or vibrating massager
- ☐ Palm pressure at temples
- ☐ Forehead/ temple rubs
- ☐ Lotion on __ arms __ legs
- ☐ Brushing or stroking hair
- ☐ Cool room temperature
- ☐ __ Loose or __ snug pajamas
- ☐ Holding pet or stuffed animal

SENSORY AREA: [Respiration / Olfactory Sense]

LUNGS

- ☐ Air purification system that filters/ cleans & ionizes
- ☐ Nasal / personal inhaler
- ☐ Other:_____
- ☐ Open nasal passages if congested (Saline spray/cool mist vaporizer)
- ☐ Walk or light exercise 1 hour+ before bedtime for 5 minutes or less
- Aromatherapy with *essential oils* to open airways & relax/ calm:
  - ☐ Eucalyptus ☐ Peppermint ☐ Tea Tree ☐ Cinnamon ☐ Lavender

SENSORY AREA: [Sight / Visual Sense]

EYES

- ☐ Picture schedule for routine
- ☐ Night light [warm tones]
- ☐ Salt Rock or Lava Lamp
- ☐ Read or look at a book
- ☐ Dimmed or rope lighting
- ☐ Corner or bed tent "womb" area
- ☐ ↓Distracters (stimulating items)
- ☐ Slow or static ceiling projection
- ☐ Other:_____

SENSORY AREA: [Hearing / Auditory Sense]

EARS

- ☐ White noise machine or fan
- ☐ Listen to a book or a CD
- ☐ Ear plugs or headphones
- ☐ Nature sounds— waterfall, ocean waves, wind, crickets, etc. (recorded or electronic)
- ☐ Classical music [< 60 beats per min.]*
- ☐ Soothing music or Metronome *
- ☐ Other:_____

SENSORY AREA: [Joints & Movement / Vestibular & Proprioceptive Sense]

POSITION

- ☐ "Womb" area- beanbag lying 30 min. before bed
- ☐ Glider rocking 30 min. prior
- ☐ Multiple sleeping bags
- ☐ Percussion on back
- ☐ Gentle rocking in bed
- ☐ Stuffed animals to hug
- ☐ Multiple bed pillows
- ☐ Calming/ Magnetic Sleep System
- ☐ Body pillow to "spoon"/hug
- ☐ Weighted blanket/ "snake"/ toys
- ☐ Other:_____

FORM C-2: SENSORY SLEEP STRATEGIES CHECKLIST (Continued)—

SENSORY AREA: [Eating or Drinking / Oral or Gustatory Sense] Period: _____ to _____

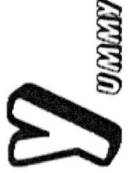

MELATONIN RICH Foods:

- ☐ Pure cherry juice
- ☐ Scottish/ Irish oatmeal* [1/2 cup for adults adolescents; 1/4 cup for children]

TRYPTOPHAN RICH Foods:

- ☐ Cottage & other cheeses
- ☐ Chew Chia seeds (2 Tbsp.)
- ☐ Peanuts/Peanut butter
- ☐ Sesame seeds/butter
- ☐ Milk—Warm or tepid
- ☐ Pineapples, plums
- ☐ Turkey patty, etc.
- ☐ Sunflower seeds
- ☐ Popcorn-Light
- ☐ Oatmeal *
- ☐ Pudding
- ☐ Yogurt
- ☐ Eggs

DETOXIFICATION AID:

- ☐ WATER—3 hours before bed & on awakening [Filtered, mineralized & Ionized—most hydrating]
- ☐ _____

DIGESTIVE AIDS:

- ☐ Cumin Seeds (↓gas, bloating & discomfort)
- ☐ Valerian Tea (sedative)
- ☐ Tilia (Tilo) Tea (calming)
- ☐ Anise Tea (gas relief)
- ☐ Chamomile Tea
- ☐ _____
- ☐ _____
- ☐ _____
- ☐ _____
- ☐ _____
- ☐ _____

OTHER CALMING FOODS:

- ☐ Bananas (↓ BP with ↑ potassium)
- ☐ Honey (glucose ↓ OREXIN that ↑ alertness)
- ☐ Non-alcoholic beer (↑ GABA, a brain tranquilizer)
- ☐ ↑ Magnesium to ↓ sweating (check with physician for levels needed)
- ☐ Cinnamon, nutmeg or vanilla (added to foods ↑ calming, muscle-relaxing alpha brain waves)
- ☐ Wheat germ (↑ Vitamin B_6)
- ☐ _____
- ☐ _____
- ☐ _____
- ☐ _____
- ☐ _____
- ☐ _____
- ☐ _____
- ☐ _____

NOTES: _____

119

Name: _____ Month: _____ Year: _____ Baseline: _____ Hours

No.	Day	Sleep Strategy*	Time Used	A M	P M	Time Asleep	A M	P M	Time Awake	A M	P M	Times Awakened	Hours Slept	IMPACT (Hours) ⇩	√ NO CHANGE	⇧
	= TOTAL NUMBER OF DAYS											TOTAL IMPACT IN HOURS:	--	+		

SUM OF IMPACT = [ ] / SUM OF DAYS = AVERAGE CHANGE: [ ]

* NOTE: Try one sensory or schedule change strategy at a time to isolate impact or effect on any possible behavioral changes.

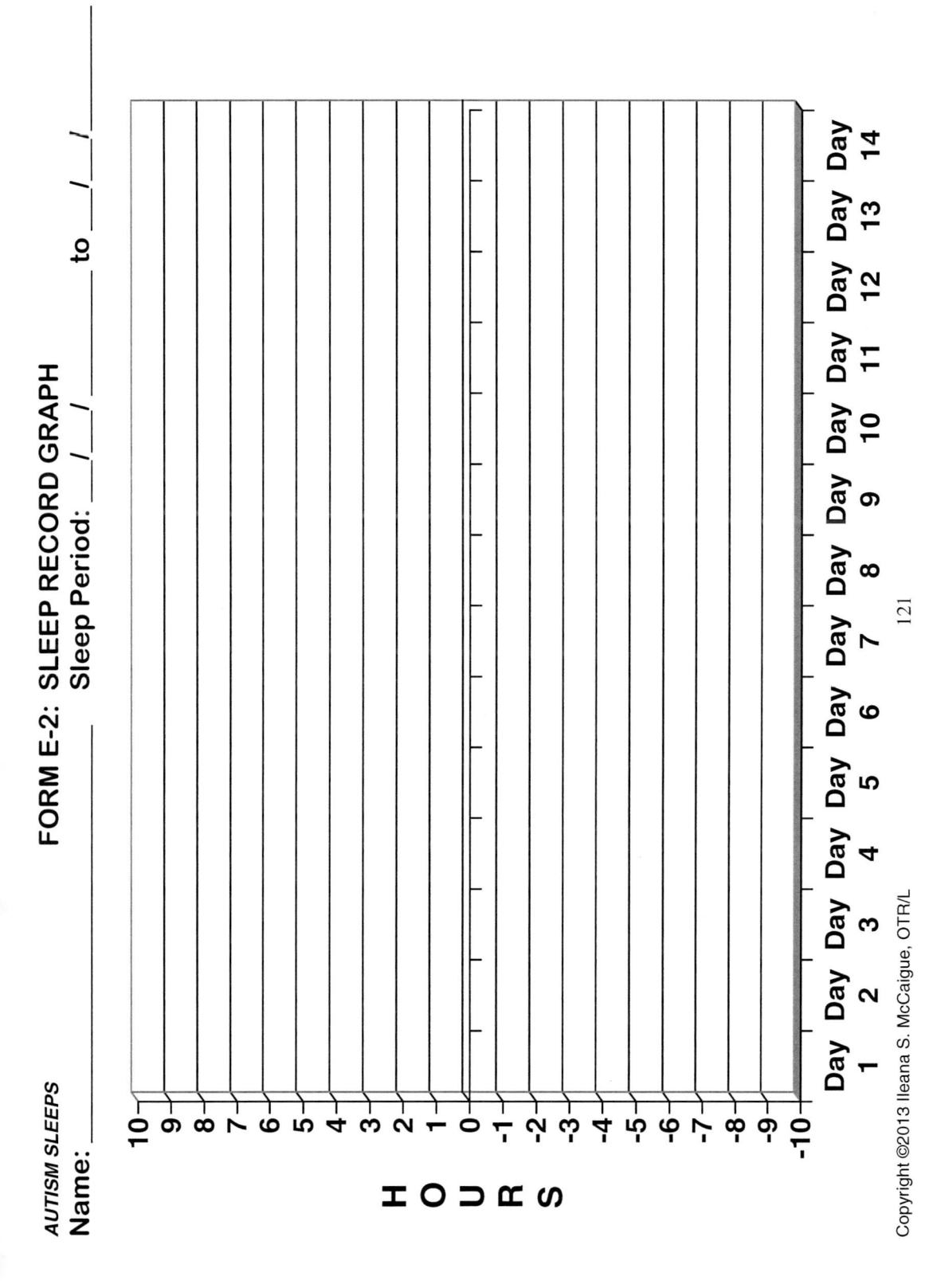

FORM A-3:   BEDTIME ROUTINE

Name: _____ Week of: __/__/_____

TIME	ACTIVITY	NOTES
	• Light snack 1 hour before bath time	
	• Take a warm water bath/shower	
	• Put on relaxing pajamas	
	• Brush teeth with warm/tepid water	
	• Go to bathroom/ potty	
	• Make room quiet & comfortable, cooler better than warmer… lights dim or off	
	• Read/look at book or listen to music/ book in "womb" area with small light	
	• Unwind ½ to 1 hour before actual bedtime using 1 or more of the following strategies: 1._____ 2._____ 3._____ 4._____	
	• Say "Good night" & leave at bedtime.	

DAY	COMMENTS	CHANGES
Monday		
Tuesday		
Wednesday		
Thursday		
Friday		
Saturday		
Sunday		

LEGEND: √ Done as listed.   Overall Reaction : + = Positive, 0 = No Impact, - = Negative

FORM B-3:   SENSORY SLEEP STRATEGIES CHECKLIST

SENSORY AREA: [Touch / Tactile Sense]   Period: _____ to _____

Skin

☐ Warm __bath or __shower 1 hour before bedtime	☐ Back rub or vibrating massager	☐ Brushing or stroking hair
	☐ Palm pressure at temples	☐ Cool room temperature
☐ Foot rub or massage	☐ Forehead/ temple rubs	☐ __Loose or __snug pajamas
☐ Face --gentle massage	☐ Lotion on __arms __legs	☐ Holding pet or stuffed animal

SENSORY AREA: [Respiration / Olfactory Sense]

Lungs

☐ Air purification system that filters/ cleans & ionizes	☐ Open nasal passages if congested (Saline spray/cool mist vaporizer) ☐ Walk or light exercise 1 hour+ before bedtime for 5 minutes or less
☐ Nasal / personal inhaler ☐ Other: _____	Aromatherapy with *essential oils* to open airways & relax/ calm: ☐ Eucalyptus ☐ Peppermint ☐ Tea Tree ☐ Cinnamon ☐ Lavender

SENSORY AREA: [Sight / Visual Sense]

Eyes

☐ Picture schedule for routine	☐ Read or look at a book	☐ ↓Distracters (stimulating items)
☐ Night light [warm tones]	☐ Dimmed or rope lighting	☐ Slow or static ceiling projection
☐ Salt Rock or Lava Lamp	☐ Corner or bed tent "womb" area	☐ Other: _____

SENSORY AREA: [Hearing / Auditory Sense]

Ears

☐ White noise machine or fan	☐ Nature sounds— waterfall, ocean waves, wind, crickets, etc. (recorded or electronic)	☐ Classical music [< 60 beats per min.]*
☐ Listen to a book or a CD		☐ Soothing music or Metronome *
☐ Ear plugs or headphones		☐ Other: _____

SENSORY AREA: [Joints & Movement / Vestibular & Proprioceptive Sense]

Position

☐ "Womb" area- beanbag lying 30 min. before bed	☐ Percussion on back	☐ Calming/ Magnetic Sleep System
☐ Glider rocking 30 min. prior	☐ Gentle rocking in bed	☐ Body pillow to "spoon"/hug
☐ Multiple sleeping bags	☐ Stuffed animals to hug	☐ Weighted blanket/ "snake"/ toys
	☐ Multiple bed pillows	☐ Other:_____

FORM C-3:   SENSORY SLEEP STRATEGIES CHECKLIST   (Continued)—

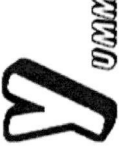

SENSORY AREA: [Eating or Drinking / Oral or Gustatory Sense] Period: _____ to _____

MELATONIN RICH Foods:

☐ Pure cherry juice

☐ Scottish/ Irish oatmeal*
[1/2 cup for adults
adolescents; 1/4 cup for
children]

TRYPTOPHAN RICH Foods:

☐ Cottage & other cheeses

☐ Chew Chia seeds (2 Tbsp.)

☐ Peanuts/Peanut butter

☐ Sesame seeds/butter

☐ Milk—Warm or tepid

☐ Pineapples, plums

☐ Turkey patty, etc.

☐ Sunflower seeds

☐ Popcorn-Light

☐ Oatmeal *

☐ Pudding

☐ Yogurt

☐ Eggs

DETOXIFICATION AID:

☐ WATER—3 hours before
bed & on awakening
[Filtered, mineralized &
Ionized—most hydrating]

☐

DIGESTIVE AIDS:

☐ Cumin Seeds (↓gas,
bloating & discomfort)

☐ Valerian Tea (sedative)

☐ Tilia (Tilo) Tea (calming)

☐ Anise Tea (gas relief)

☐ Chamomile Tea

☐

☐

☐

☐

☐

☐

OTHER CALMING FOODS:

☐ Bananas (↓ BP with ↑ potassium)

☐ Honey (glucose ↓ OREXIN that ↑
alertness)

☐ Non-alcoholic beer (↑ GABA, a brain
tranquilizer)

☐ ↑ Magnesium to ↓ sweating (check
with physician for levels needed)

☐ Cinnamon, nutmeg or vanilla (added to
foods ↑ calming, muscle-relaxing
alpha brain waves)

☐ Wheat germ (↑ Vitamin B_6)

☐

☐

☐

☐

☐

☐

☐

NOTES: _____

FORM D-3: SLEEP RECORD

Page ___

Name: _____ Month: _____ Year:_____ Baseline: _____ Hours

No.	Day	Sleep Strategy*	Time Used	A M	P M	Time Asleep	A M	P M	Time Awake	A M	P M	Times Awakened	Hours Slept	IMPACT (Hours) ⇩	√ NO CHANGE	⇧

	= TOTAL NUMBER OF DAYS			TOTAL IMPACT IN HOURS:	--	+

SUM OF IMPACT = [ ] / SUM OF DAYS = AVERAGE CHANGE: [ ]

NOTE: Try one sensory or schedule change strategy at a time to isolate impact or effect on any possible behavioral changes.

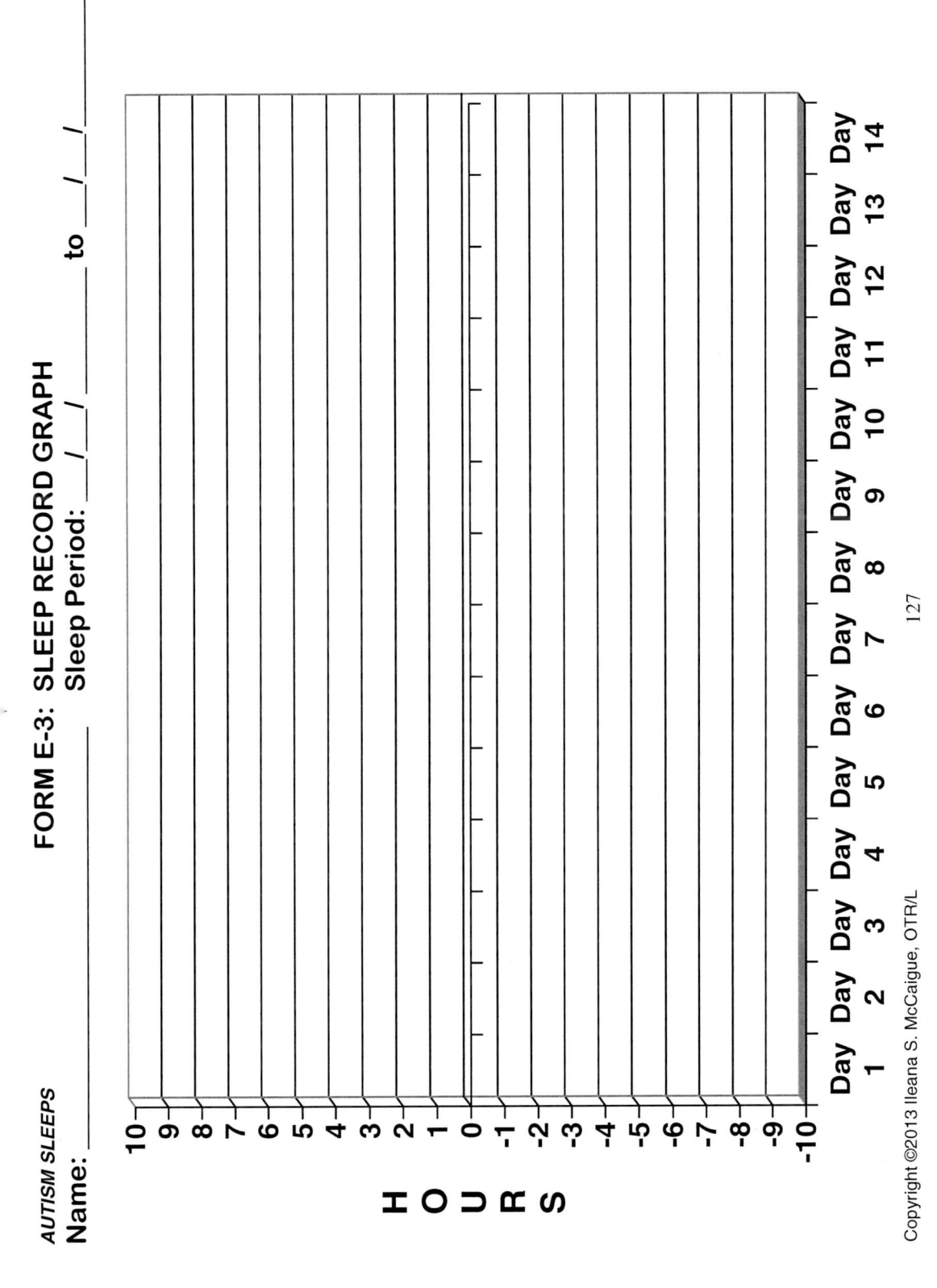

AUTISM SLEEPS

FORM E-3: SLEEP RECORD GRAPH

Name: _____

Sleep Period: ___ / ___ / ___ to ___ / ___ / ___

FORM A-4:   BEDTIME ROUTINE

Name: _____ Week of: __/__/_____

TIME	ACTIVITY	NOTES
	• Light snack 1 hour before bath time	
	• Take a warm water bath/shower	
	• Put on relaxing pajamas	
	• Brush teeth with warm/tepid water	
	• Go to bathroom/ potty	
	• Make room quiet & comfortable, cooler better than warmer... lights dim or off	
	• Read/look at book or listen to music/ book in "womb" area with small light	
	• Unwind ½ to 1 hour before actual bedtime using 1 or more of the following strategies: 1._____ 2._____ 3._____ 4._____	
	• Say "Good night" & leave at bedtime.	

DAY	COMMENTS	CHANGES
Monday		
Tuesday		
Wednesday		
Thursday		
Friday		
Saturday		
Sunday		

LEGEND: √ Done as listed.   Overall Reaction : + = Positive, 0 = No Impact, - = Negative

SENSORY SLEEP STRATEGIES CHECKLIST

Period: _____ to _____

SENSORY AREA: [Touch / Tactile Sense]

☐ Warm __bath or __shower 1 hour before bedtime
☐ Foot rub or massage
☐ Face --gentle massage

☐ Back rub or vibrating massager
☐ Palm pressure at temples
☐ Forehead/ temple rubs
☐ Lotion on __arms __legs

☐ Brushing or stroking hair
☐ Cool room temperature
☐ __Loose or __ snug pajamas
☐ Holding pet or stuffed animal

SENSORY AREA: [Respiration / Olfactory Sense]

☐ Air purification system that filters/ cleans & ionizes
☐ Nasal / personal inhaler
☐ Other: _____

☐ Open nasal passages if congested (Saline spray/cool mist vaporizer)
☐ Walk or light exercise 1 hour+ before bedtime for 5 minutes or less

Aromatherapy with *essential oils* to open airways & relax/ calm:
☐ Eucalyptus ☐ Peppermint ☐ Tea Tree ☐ Cinnamon ☐ Lavender

SENSORY AREA: [Sight / Visual Sense]

☐ Picture schedule for routine
☐ Night light [warm tones]
☐ Salt Rock or Lava Lamp

☐ Read or look at a book
☐ Dimmed or rope lighting
☐ Corner or bed tent "womb" area

☐ ↓Distracters (stimulating items)
☐ Slow or static ceiling projection
☐ Other: _____

SENSORY AREA: [Hearing / Auditory Sense]

☐ White noise machine or fan
☐ Listen to a book or a CD
☐ Ear plugs or headphones

☐ Nature sounds— waterfall, ocean waves, wind, crickets, etc. (recorded or electronic)

☐ Classical music [< 60 beats per min.]*
☐ Soothing music or Metronome *
☐ Other: _____

SENSORY AREA: [Joints & Movement / Vestibular & Proprioceptive Sense]

☐ "Womb" area- beanbag lying 30 min. before bed
☐ Glider rocking 30 min. prior
☐ Multiple sleeping bags

☐ Percussion on back
☐ Gentle rocking in bed
☐ Stuffed animals to hug
☐ Multiple bed pillows

☐ Calming/ Magnetic Sleep System
☐ Body pillow to "spoon"/hug
☐ Weighted blanket/ "snake"/ toys
☐ Other: _____

S KIN

L UNGS

E YES

E ARS

P OSITION

FORM C-4:   SENSORY SLEEP STRATEGIES CHECKLIST   (Continued)—

SENSORY AREA: [Eating or Drinking / Oral or Gustatory Sense] Period: _____ to _____

Yummy

MELATONIN RICH Foods:	DETOXIFICATION AID:	OTHER CALMING FOODS:
□ Pure cherry juice	□ WATER—3 hours before bed & on awakening	□ Bananas ($\downarrow$ BP with $\uparrow$ potassium)
□ Scottish/ Irish oatmeal* [1/2 cup for adults adolescents; 1/4 cup for children]	[Filtered, mineralized & Ionized—most hydrating]	□ Honey (glucose $\downarrow$ OREXIN that $\uparrow$ alertness)
	□ _____	□ Non-alcoholic beer ($\uparrow$ GABA, a brain tranquilizer)
TRYPTOPHAN RICH Foods:	**DIGESTIVE AIDS:**	□ $\uparrow$ Magnesium to $\downarrow$ sweating (check with physician for levels needed)
□ Cottage & other cheeses	□ Cumin Seeds ($\downarrow$gas, bloating & discomfort)	
□ Chew Chia seeds (2 Tbsp.)		□ Cinnamon, nutmeg or vanilla (added to foods $\uparrow$ calming, muscle-relaxing alpha brain waves)
□ Peanuts/Peanut butter	□ Valerian Tea (sedative)	
□ Sesame seeds/butter	□ Tilia (Tilo) Tea (calming)	
□ Milk—Warm or tepid	□ Anise Tea (gas relief)	□ Wheat germ ($\uparrow$ Vitamin B_6)
□ Pineapples, plums	□ Chamomile Tea	□ _____
□ Turkey patty, etc.	□ _____	□ _____
□ Sunflower seeds	□ _____	□ _____
□ Popcorn-Light	□ _____	□ _____
□ Oatmeal *	□ _____	□ _____
□ Pudding	□ _____	□ _____
□ Yogurt	□ _____	□ _____
□ Eggs		

NOTES: _____

_____

_____

_____

AUTISM SLEEPS   FORM D-4: SLEEP RECORD   Page ___

Name: _____   Month: _____ Year:_____   Baseline: _____ Hours

No.	Day	Sleep Strategy*	Time Used	A M	P M	Time Asleep	A M	P M	Time Awake	A M	P M	Times Awakened	Hours Slept	IMPACT (Hours) ⇩	√ NO CHANGE	⇧

| | = TOTAL NUMBER OF DAYS | | | | | | | | | TOTAL IMPACT IN HOURS: | -- | + |

SUM OF IMPACT = [ ]   / SUM OF DAYS = AVERAGE CHANGE: [ ]

NOTE: Try one sensory or schedule change strategy at a time to isolate impact or effect on any possible behavioral changes.

FORM E-4: SLEEP RECORD GRAPH

Name: _____

Sleep Period: ___/___/_____ to ___/___/_____

H
O
U
R
S

10
9
8
7
6
5
4
3
2
1
0
-1
-2
-3
-4
-5
-6
-7
-8
-9
-10

Day 1 Day 2 Day 3 Day 4 Day 5 Day 6 Day 7 Day 8 Day 9 Day 10 Day 11 Day 12 Day 13 Day 14

133

FORM A-5:   BEDTIME ROUTINE

Name: _____ Week of: __/__/____

TIME	ACTIVITY	NOTES
	• Light snack 1 hour before bath time	
	• Take a warm water bath/shower	
	• Put on relaxing pajamas	
	• Brush teeth with warm/tepid water	
	• Go to bathroom/potty	
	• Make room quiet & comfortable, cooler better than warmer… lights dim or off	
	• Read/look at book or listen to music/ book in "womb" area with small light	
	• Unwind ½ to 1 hour before actual bedtime using 1 or more of the following strategies: 1._____ 2._____ 3._____ 4._____	
	• Say "Good night" & leave at bedtime.	

DAY	COMMENTS	CHANGES
Monday		
Tuesday		
Wednesday		
Thursday		
Friday		
Saturday		
Sunday		

LEGEND: √ Done as listed.   Overall Reaction : + = Positive, 0 = No Impact, - = Negative

FORM B-5: SENSORY SLEEP STRATEGIES CHECKLIST

Period: _____ to _____

SENSORY AREA: [Touch / Tactile Sense]

- ☐ Warm __ bath or __ shower 1 hour before bedtime
- ☐ Foot rub or massage
- ☐ Face --gentle massage

- ☐ Back rub or vibrating massager
- ☐ Palm pressure at temples
- ☐ Forehead/ temple rubs
- ☐ Lotion on __ arms __ legs

- ☐ Brushing or stroking hair
- ☐ Cool room temperature
- ☐ __ Loose or __ snug pajamas
- ☐ Holding pet or stuffed animal

SENSORY AREA: [Respiration / Olfactory Sense]

- ☐ Air purification system that filters/ cleans & ionizes
- ☐ Nasal / personal inhaler
- ☐ Other: _____

- ☐ Open nasal passages if congested (Saline spray/cool mist vaporizer)
- ☐ Walk or light exercise 1 hour+ before bedtime for 5 minutes or less

Aromatherapy with *essential oils* to open airways & relax/ calm:
- ☐ Eucalyptus ☐ Peppermint ☐ Tea Tree ☐ Cinnamon ☐ Lavender

SENSORY AREA: [Sight / Visual Sense]

- ☐ Picture schedule for routine
- ☐ Night light [warm tones]
- ☐ Salt Rock or Lava Lamp

- ☐ Read or look at a book
- ☐ Dimmed or rope lighting
- ☐ Corner or bed tent "womb" area

- ☐ ↓Distracters (stimulating items)
- ☐ Slow or static ceiling projection
- ☐ Other: _____

SENSORY AREA: [Hearing / Auditory Sense]

- ☐ White noise machine or fan
- ☐ Listen to a book or a CD
- ☐ Ear plugs or headphones

- ☐ Nature sounds— waterfall, ocean waves, wind, crickets, etc. (recorded or electronic)

- ☐ Classical music [< 60 beats per min.]*
- ☐ Soothing music or Metronome *
- ☐ Other: _____

SENSORY AREA: [Joints & Movement / Vestibular & Proprioceptive Sense]

- ☐ "Womb" area- beanbag lying 30 min. before bed
- ☐ Glider rocking 30 min. prior
- ☐ Multiple sleeping bags

- ☐ Percussion on back
- ☐ Gentle rocking in bed
- ☐ Stuffed animals to hug
- ☐ Multiple bed pillows

- ☐ Calming/ Magnetic Sleep System
- ☐ Body pillow to "spoon"/hug
- ☐ Weighted blanket/ "snake"/ toys
- ☐ Other: _____

S KIN
L UNGS
E YES
E ARS
P OSITION

FORM C-5: SENSORY SLEEP STRATEGIES CHECKLIST (Continued)—

SENSORY AREA: [Eating or Drinking / Oral or Gustatory Sense] Period: _____ to _____

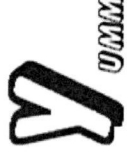

MELATONIN RICH Foods:

☐ Pure cherry juice
☐ Scottish/ Irish oatmeal*
[1/2 cup for adults
adolescents; 1/4 cup for
children]

TRYPTOPHAN RICH Foods:

☐ Cottage & other cheeses
☐ Chew Chia seeds (2 Tbsp.)
☐ Peanuts/Peanut butter
☐ Sesame seeds/butter
☐ Milk—Warm or tepid
☐ Pineapples, plums
☐ Turkey patty, etc.
☐ Sunflower seeds
☐ Popcorn–Light
☐ Oatmeal *
☐ Pudding
☐ Yogurt
☐ Eggs

DETOXIFICATION AID:

☐ WATER—3 hours before
bed & on awakening
[Filtered, mineralized &
Ionized—most hydrating]
☐ _____

DIGESTIVE AIDS:

☐ Cumin Seeds (↓gas,
bloating & discomfort)
☐ Valerian Tea (sedative)
☐ Tilia (Tilo) Tea (calming)
☐ Anise Tea (gas relief)
☐ Chamomile Tea
☐ _____
☐ _____
☐ _____
☐ _____

OTHER CALMING FOODS:

☐ Bananas (↓ BP with ↑ potassium)
☐ Honey (glucose ↓ OREXIN that ↑
alertness)
☐ Non-alcoholic beer (↑ GABA, a brain
tranquilizer)
☐ ↑ Magnesium to ↓ sweating (check
with physician for levels needed)
☐ Cinnamon, nutmeg or vanilla (added to
foods ↑ calming, muscle-relaxing
alpha brain waves)
☐ Wheat germ (↑ Vitamin B_6)
☐ _____
☐ _____
☐ _____
☐ _____
☐ _____
☐ _____
☐ _____
☐ _____

NOTES: _____

_____

_____

_____

_____

Name: _____   Month: _____ Year:_____   Baseline: _____ Hours

No.	Day	Sleep Strategy*	Time Used	A M	P M	Time Asleep	A M	P M	Time Awake	A M	P M	Times Awakened	Hours Slept	IMPACT (Hours) ⇩	√ NO CHANGE	⇧
	= TOTAL NUMBER OF DAYS											TOTAL IMPACT IN HOURS:		--	+

SUM OF IMPACT = [   ]   / SUM OF DAYS = AVERAGE CHANGE: [   ]

NOTE: Try one sensory or schedule change strategy at a time to isolate impact or effect on any possible behavioral changes.

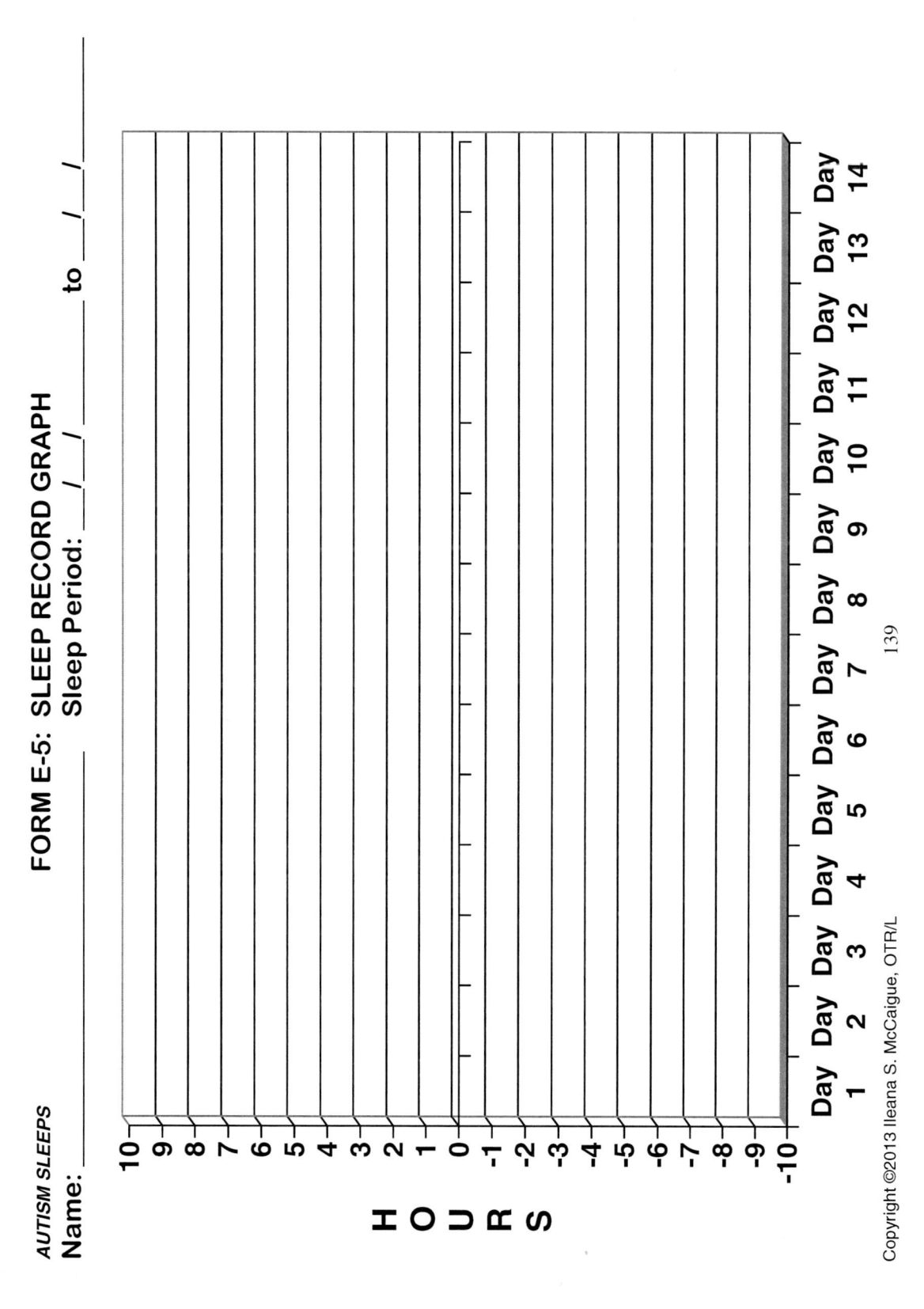

AUTISM SLEEPS

FORM E-5: SLEEP RECORD GRAPH

Name: _____

Sleep Period: ___/___/___ to ___/___/___

HOURS

10
9
8
7
6
5
4
3
2
1
0
-1
-2
-3
-4
-5
-6
-7
-8
-9
-10

Day 1 Day 2 Day 3 Day 4 Day 5 Day 6 Day 7 Day 8 Day 9 Day 10 Day 11 Day 12 Day 13 Day 14

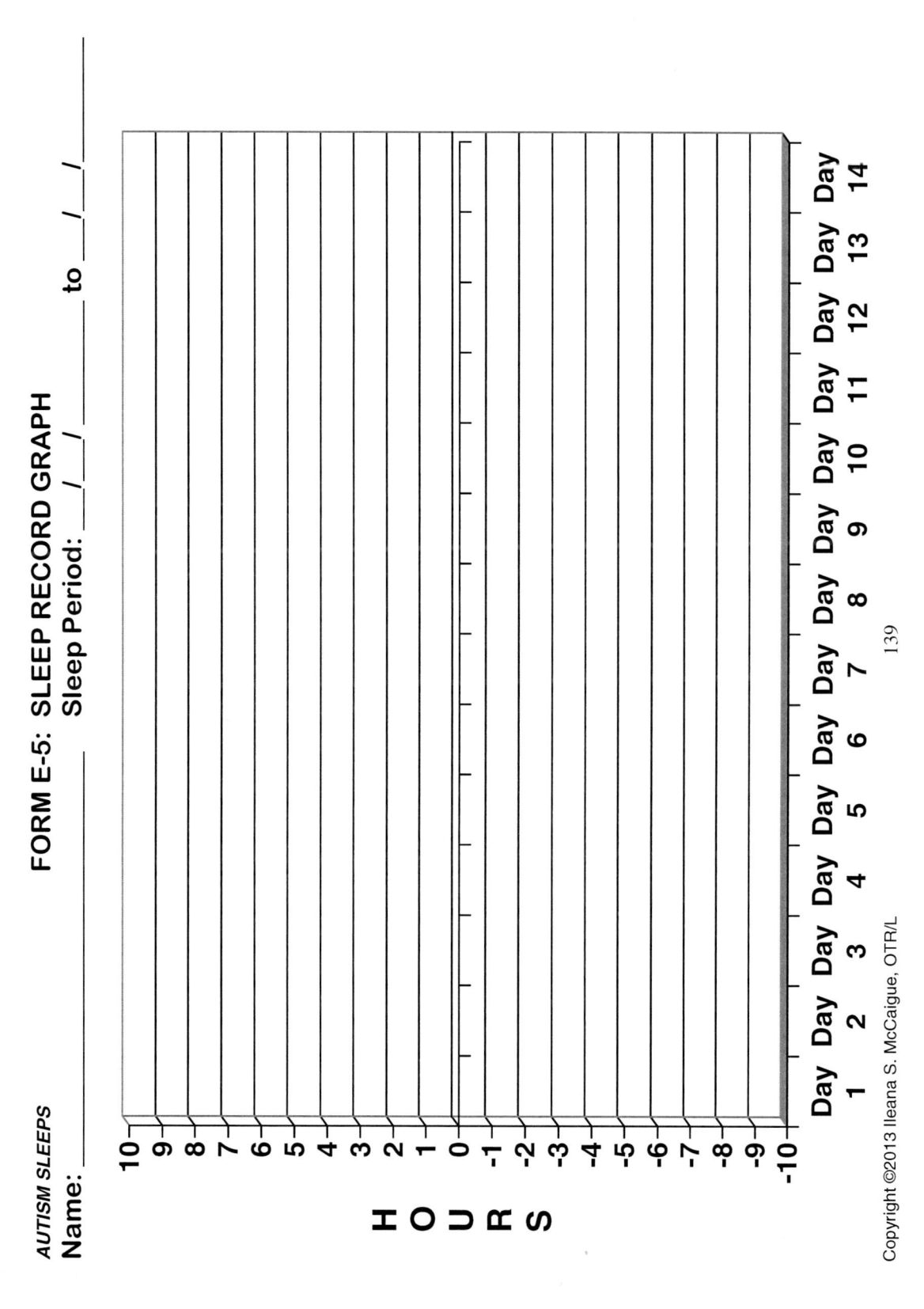

139

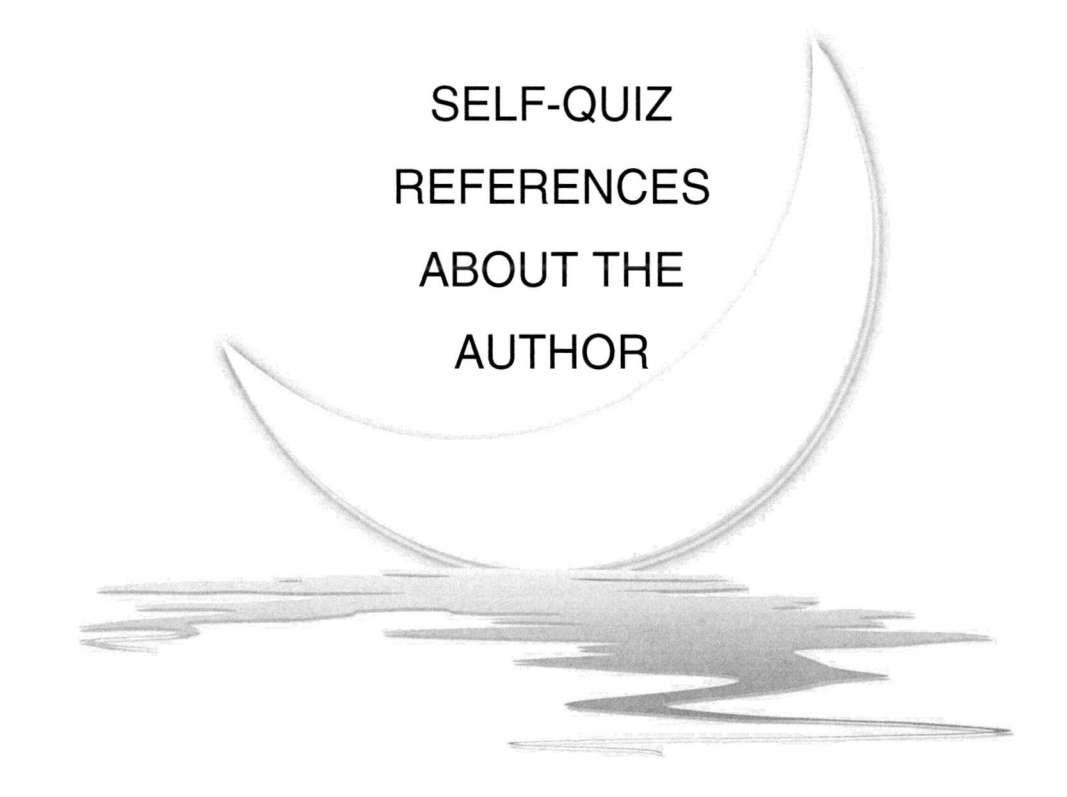

SELF-QUIZ

REFERENCES

ABOUT THE

AUTHOR

SELF QUIZ: Post-Test Questions

Name: _____   Date: _____

1. When do most children give up taking a nap?
   a. 2 years
   b. 3 years
   c. 4 years
   d. 5 years

2. Which of the following might interfere with a child sleeping through the night?
   a. falling asleep with a bottle
   b. falling asleep on the couch and then being moved to the bed
   c. falling asleep while watching TV
   d. all of the above

3. A good security object in bed as part of the routine could include a…
   a. blanket
   b. bottle of juice or milk
   c. stuffed animal
   d. either a or c

4. How much sleep does a 3-month-old usually need?
   a. 20 hours
   b. 15 hours
   c. 12 hours
   d.   9 hours

5. How much sleep does a 9-year-old need?
   a. 12 hours
   b. 11 hours
   c. 10 hours
   d.   9 hours

[CONTINUED ON NEXT PAGE]

SELF-QUIZ: Post-Test Questions (Continued)-

Name: _____ Date: _____

6. How much sleep does a 2-year-old usually need?
   a. 15 hours
   b. 13 hours
   c. 11 hours
   d. 9 hours

7. How much sleep does a 14-year-old need?
   a. 11 hours
   b. 10 hours
   c. 9 hours
   d. 8 hours

8. How much sleep does a 5-year-old need?
   a. 15 hours
   b. 13 hours
   c. 11 hours
   d. 9 hours

9. Children with obstructive sleep apnea usually…
   a. snore
   b. snore loudly and have periods where they stop breathing
   c. are thin
   d. have had their tonsils taken out

10. Not getting enough sleep at night can cause children to…
    a. have trouble paying attention
    b. have headaches
    c. be hyperactive
    d. all of the above

[END OF TEST]

POST-TEST SCORE: _____% Correct   CHANGE: + / - _____%

ANSWERS TO SELF-QUIZ

1. d. 5 years

2. d. All of the above

3. d. Either a. or c.

4. b. 15 hours

5. c. 10 hours

6. b. 13 hours

7. c. 9 hours

8. c. 11 hours

9. b. Snore loudly and have periods

   where they stop breathing

10. d. All of the above

REFERENCES

BOOKS

- I. S. McCaigue, OTR/L, CDRS, *The Scale of Sensory Strategies (S.O.S.S.) Toolkit™*, Handy O.T. Treatment Tools, Georgia (2010).

- C. H. Schenck, MD, *Sleep—A Groundbreaking Guide to the Mysteries, the Problems, and the Solutions*, Avery—The Penguin Group, New York (2008); pp.1-12.

- V. G. Cooksley, R.N., *Aromatherapy—Soothing Remedies to Restore, Rejuvenate, and Heal*, Prentice Hall Press, New York (2002); pp. 213-218.

- D. Hales, *An Invitation to Health*, 6th Edition, The Benjamin/Cummings Publishing Company, Inc., New York (1994); pp. 64-66.

- M. Walker, *The Power of Color* (1991), by L. Barker.

WEBSITES

- *About.com*, Pediatrics, "Kids and Bedtime Routines."

- *About.com*, Pediatrics, "Children's Sleep Quiz."

- *About.com*, Pediatrics, "Guide Picks-Top 10 Sleep Parenting Books."

- *About.com*, Single Parents, "A Bedtime Routine That Works."

- *Circadiandisorders.org,* Canadian Sleep Disorders Association

- *ClinicalTrials.gov*, "Treatment of Sleep Problems in Children With Autism Spectrum Disorder With Melatonin (REST)."

- *Djreprints.com*, "Grown-Up Problems Start at Bedtime."

- *DoctorOz.com*. Dr. Pina LoGiudice, ND, on show on July 16, 2012

- FunandFunction.com

- FutureHorizons.com

REFERENCES (Continued)-

WEBSITES

- *HOTRxTools.com (Products Tab for Wellness)* Sensory Tools for Healthy Living

- *NIKKEN.com/SENSORYTOOLS4U*

- *SchoolSpecialty.com*

- *Sleepforkids.org*, "Children and Sleep."

- *Sleepsense.net/do-it-yourself-options*, Dana Obleman's, "The Sleep Sense Program".

- *SpiffyMoms.com*, "Bedtime Tips for Special Needs Kids," Therapro.com

- *TherapyShoppe.com*

- *WebMD.com*, "Helping Your Child With Autism Get a Good Night's Sleep".

- *WebMD.com/sleep-disorders/guide/sleephygiene*, Sleep Disorders Health Center, "How to Sleep Better".

- *WebMD.com*, "Put Sleep Difficulties to Bed: Advice for Parents of Children with Autism."

- *WebMD.com/sleepdisorders/guide/sleep-hygiene*, Sleep Disorders Health Center, "Understanding Sleep Problems—the Basics."

- *Webmetronome.com*

- *WhiteNoisePlayer.com*

- *YourTherapySource.com*

CREDITS

- CLIP ART: Microsoft Office

REFERENCES (Continued)-

CREDITS

- GRAPHIC p. 65: Monster; Vickie A. Johnson, Ed.S.; President, North Gwinnett Arts Association (*president@ngaa4arts.com*); *vsjohnsonperceptions@charter.net*

- ILLUSTRATION p. 14: "Effects of sleep deprivation" by Mikael Häggström, MD. The image is made available under the Creative Commons CC0 1.0 Universal Public Domain Dedication; *http://en.wikipedia.org/Wiki/File:Effects_of_sleep_deprivation .svg#Summary*

- ILLUSTRATION p. 55: Sleeping Positions; Nurinda Qhiqy Rachmawati; *nurindaqhiqy @gmail.com*

- ILLUSTRATION p. 104: Bedtime Chart; *www.FreePrintableBehaviorCharts.com*

- PHOTOS pp. 37, 55, 56, 62: Hearing Protectors, Vibrasonic Massage Brush, Sensation Vibration Pillows, Hand-Held Massager, Relaxation Center Indoor Tent; School Specialty, Inc.; *www.Abilitations.com*

- PHOTO p. 38: B-Calm Audio System; B-Calm, LLC; *www.b-calmsound.com*

- PHOTO pp. 38: Relaxation CD for Children-"A Moment of Peace"; Best You Can Be Foundation; Debbie Milam; *www.bestyoucanbe.org*

- PHOTOS pp. 38, 45, 55, 56, 60, 61: "Cool Bananas" CD, Set of 30 Sensory Stories on CD, Super Chews, Wilbarger-Therapressure Brushes, Thera-Band Hand Exercise Balls, Corner Sensory Bundle; Therapro, Inc.; *www.therapro.com*

- PHOTOS pp. 38: Sleep Sheep; Cloud•b; *www.Cloudb.com*

- PHOTOS p. 39: Visual Timers; Jan Rogers; Time Timer, LLC; *www.timetimer.com*

- PHOTOS pp. 41, 51, 56, 61, 62: Sleep Mask, Mag Creator, Mag Duo, SPORT Water Bottle, PiMag Waterfall System, Magnetic Sleep System (mattress topper, pillow, comforter), KenkoLight II; *www.Nikken.com/SensoryTools4U*

- PHOTO p. 42: Insomnia Relief personal inhaler; Dr. David Epstein, D.O.; Earth Solutions; *www.earthsolutions.com*

REFERENCES (Continued)-

CREDITS

- PHOTO p. 42: Wyndmere Electric Diffuser, MIO Personal Diffuser, Scent Ball; *www.Wyndmerenaturals.com*

- PHOTOS p. 45: Z-Vibe, Z-Grabber; *Rebecca Lowsky, rebecca.lowsky@gmail.com*

- PHOTO p. 45: Chewy Tube; Speech Pathology Associates, LLC; *cushingjw@aol.com*

- PHOTOS p. 55: Weighted blanket, sleeping bag; *FunandFunction.com*

- PHOTO p. 58: Airwalker suspended swing; Dye-namic Movement Products, sensory movement tools; *www.dyenamicmovement.com*

- PHOTO p. 60: Getting Ready for Bed book; Sandbox Learning Company; *www.sandbox-learning.com*

- PHOTO p. 61: Projecting Constellation Turtle; Hammacher Schlemmer; *www.hammacher.com*

- PHOTO p. 62: Bed Tents for boys and girls; Pacific Play Tents, Inc.; *www.pacific playtents.com*

- PHOTOS p. 64, 65: Ms. Stephanie's Potions, Stuffies; Stephanie Corey; *www.Miss StephaniesPotions.com*

- PHOTOS, STOCK: Dreamstime, *www.dreamstime.com*; iStockphoto, *www.istock photo.com*

ABOUT THE AUTHOR
Ileana S. McCaigue, OTR/L

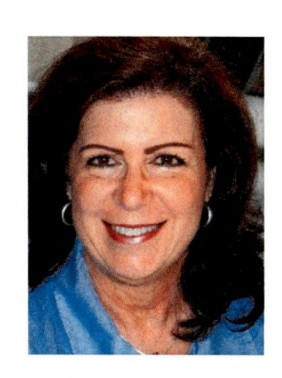

A 1977 summa cum laude graduate from the Medical College of Georgia in Augusta, Georgia, Ileana is an Occupational Therapist with over 36 years of experience in the field of Occupational Therapy. She is nationally certified/registered, licensed by the state of Georgia, and has specialty certifications in Sensory Integration, as a past Certified Driver Rehabilitation Specialist, and for use of the Interactive Metronome to evaluate and treat sensory processing disorders. She was also trained in Active Parenting techniques.

Ileana has served as an expert witness for cases involving infants and children, and is a published author. Having presented in-services, seminars and workshops nationally throughout her career, Ileana is an experienced speaker. She has covered subject matters from the Neonatal Intensive Care Unit to pediatric concerns in the home, school and community, especially with regards to sensory strategy implementation for a variety of sensory-based behavioral concerns.

Ileana was the recipient in October 2005 of the Barbara S. Grant Award from the Georgia O.T. Association for her dedication and lifetime of outstanding service to the field of occupational therapy. In 1977 she received the Maddak Award in the area of Physical Disability for the design of the *S.K.A.T.E.* (Skateboard for Kinesthetic Arm Therapeutic Exercises) .

Since 1995 Ileana has worked in a metro Atlanta area public school system. She works with special needs students in the elementary, middle and high schools within the Special Education Department that require Related Services to provide direct and consultative support to teachers and students to help meet Individualized Education Plan objectives.

ABOUT THE AUTHOR   (Continued)-
Ileana S. McCaigue, OTR/L

She sees private clients to provide home and community-based treatment as needed, including pre-driving assessments, sensory-integration therapy, Interactive Metronome and other sensory and brain-based interventions. Her specialty lies in the areas of children, adolescents and adults with Sensory Processing Disorders, especially those involved in Autism Spectrum Disorders, Attention Deficit Hyperactivity Disorders, and Specific Learning Disabilities that have sensory-based problem behaviors.

In addition to her Occupational Therapy practice, she has promoted the therapeutic use of magnets and other essential elements that helped her recovery after a significant back injury in 1998. She provides free consultations regarding the use of wellness products, and has been an independent NIKKEN wellness consultant since 2010. After her near fatal auto accident in 2002, where she was hit directly on her driver's side at the speed of 85 miles per hour, she did her own rehabilitation and fully recovered from a pelvic fracture, Colles fracture of her left forearm and a mild head injury where she regained her short-term memory after nine months. She used holistic products and natural methods to help her body and brain heal itself without the need for surgery. She promotes these and other products that provide *Sensory Tools for Healthy Living* with sensory strategies to help balance lifestyles and enable individuals to live healthier lives through her website: *www.NIKKEN.com/SensoryTools4U.*

Ileana is the proud mother of a son who is a graduate of the University of Georgia, and a daughter who is an honors graduate of Kennesaw State University. She was born in Havana, Cuba, and immigrated into the United States in 1957. She is bilingual and fluent in Spanish, her native language. She is also involved in her community doing a variety of volunteer work as a graduate of the Suwanee Citizens Police Academy; serves on the Board of the Friends of Suwanee Police Department; does animal-assisted therapy with her sweet Shorkie, Katie; and is a photographer and member of the North Gwinnett Arts Association.

NOTES:

NOTES: